PRACTICAL GERIATRIC ASSESSMENT

PRACTICAL GERIATRIC ASSESSMENT

HOWARD M. FILLIT, MD

Corporate Medical Director For Medicare
Corporate Medical Affairs
NYLCare Health Plans, Inc.
New York, NY
And
Clinical Professor Of Geriatrics And Medicine
The Henry L. Schwartz Department Of Geriatrics And Adult Development
The Mount Sinai Medical Center
New York, NY

and

GLORIA PICARIELLO, MSN, RN, CS

Manager, Geriatric Care Services
Corporate Medical Affairs
NYLCare Health Plans, Inc.
New York, NY

Greenwich Medical Media Ltd
219 The Linen Hall
162-168 Regent Street
London
W1R 5TB

ISBN: 1 900 151 901

First Published 1998

A catalogue record for this book is available from the British Library.

Distributed worldwide by
Oxford University Press

Designed and Produced by
Diane Parker, Saldatore Limited

Printed in Great Britain by
Ashford Colour Press

Foreward
by Robert N. Butler, M.D.
Professor of Geriatrics
Director, International Longevity Center (US).
Department of Geriatrics & Adult Development, The Mount Sinai Medical Center

While a member of the nation's first medical school department of geriatrics, Dr. Howard Fillit inaugurated one of the first multipurpose acute care geriatrics units in a non-veterans hospital setting. On the basis of his experience and with the support of the Sandoz Pharmaceutical Company, he developed *A Practical Guide for Geriatric Assessment* in 1990. He has now greatly expanded this practical guide to geriatric assessment in terms of both scope and application. This reorganization particularly focuses upon primary care in the ambulatory setting. He has added the important voice of nursing with his co-author, Gloria Picariello. Both authors have had many years of experience in the primary care practice of geriatrics and in Medicare managed care.

The world is growing older, given the revolutionary increase in longevity. Simultaneously, there is considerable reorganization of health care in the industrialized world. In the United States in particular, managed care is beginning to take hold. Obviously, this book is exceptionally useful to those who practice in managed care settings where every effort must be made to enhance quality as well as efficacy of care. The book will be of use to all physicians, nurses, social workers, and other health professionals involved in the practice of geriatrics. The first edition was well received, and this larger and reorganized version will be even more popular

Preface

This practical guide for geriatric assessment began as a project initiated in 1990 which led to the first version for application primarily in the acute care setting. The initial version was published in monograph form in a limited printing which received numerous requests (Fillit, H.M.,1994, *A Practical Guide to Geriatric Assessment,* monograph, Sandoz Corporation, Basle, Switzerland). As a result, the current text was created to expand on the original both in terms of scope and application. The text has been reorganized for the practice of geriatric assessment in any setting, but particularly with a focus on the primary care, ambulatory setting.

The current text is now the result of the cumulative knowledge of both authors' many years of experience in the primary care practice of geriatrics and in Medicare managed care. It is not just fortunate that the text is co-authored by a geriatrician and a geriatric nurse practitioner. This is representative of the multidisciplinary nature of geriatric practice and indicates that the book can and should be employed by physicians, nurses, social workers and other health care professionals involved in the practice of geriatrics.

Throughout the world, extraordinary changes in the organization of health care are occuring, with managed care now practically the norm in most of the United States. At the same time, the geriatric imperative is placing demands on health systems with growing populations of elderly individuals with unique needs. These demographic and organizational changes in the health care system have created an increasing need for guides like this one which can facilitate the process of geriatric assessment.

However, ultimately it is our desire to promote the quality of geriatric care. The geriatric patient is highly complex. Organization is a crucial skill in the care of the geriatric patient, especially in a world of managed care. We like to say that "geriatric assessment is a verb, not a noun." It is a process that promotes comprehensive and efficient care for complex frail elderly patients. The purpose of this book is to provide the clinical practitioner in geriatrics with a guide, a method, and specific, generally validated "instruments" to make the process of geriatric assessment both comprehensive and efficient. Some instruments have been adapted from previously published articles. In these cases, the original references are cited. In other cases where no assessment instrument previously existed, we have tried to create one. While our own instruments may not have scientifically demonstrated predictive validity, the "instruments" represent our own knowledge of what is required to assess the patient for a particular syndrome.

We are both grateful to NYLCare Health Plans, Inc., and particularly to Samuel Warburton, MD, Senior Vice President for Medical Affairs and Chief Medical Officer, for their commitment to quality geriatric care, and providing the support for our work on this text. However, the text in no way represents any official policies or procedures of NYLCare and is solely the opinions of the authors.

Howard M. Fillitt, MD   Gloria Picariello, MSN, RN, CS

TABLE OF CONTENTS

PART I. COMPREHENSIVE GERIATRIC ASSESSMENT: AN OVERVIEW

COMPREHENSIVE GERIATRIC ASSESSMENT: AN OVERVIEW

Introduction

It is estimated that the US elderly population will grow from 25.5 million in 1980 to a projected 64.3 million in 2030, a doubling of this group in 50 years. Individuals over the age of 75 years are the most rapidly growing segment of the overall elderly population. The health problems of individuals over the age of 75 years are generally characterized by a multiplicity of chronic, progressive, generally incurable medical illnesses which are associated with significant mental health, functional health, and social health problems. As a result, health care for these individuals focuses not on cure, but rather on the maintenance of functional health. Effective, humane and efficient chronic care management is the hallmark of quality geriatric care.

The Target Population for Geriatric Assessment — The Frail Elderly

High risk seniors are characterized as the "frail" elderly. The *frail elderly* are the **target** population of geriatric assessment and care management programs. Recognition and understanding of the frail elderly as the target population of this program are critical to its success. The *frail elderly* are individuals, generally over the age of 75 years, who suffer complex, multidiscplinary health problems. The frail elderly are functionally impaired, and their health problems are generally complicated by significant psychosocial impairments, including mental health problems such as dementia or depression, as well as social isolation and poverty. As a result of the multidisciplinary nature of their health problems, the frail elderly require high risk identification and a multidisciplinary geriatric team to provide quality and efficient health care.

The frail elderly are readily distinguishable from the well elderly who may suffer from one or two "mild" chronic illnesses which are manageable, and who are not functionally impaired and are living independently. The frail elderly can be readily and clearly identified by high risk screening.

Promotion and maintenance of *functional independence* to the highest degree that is reasonably possible is the primary goal of geriatric care, maintaining individuals at the site of maximum functional independence (for example living independently at home), preventing hospitalization and institutionalization. These goals can be achieved by quality and efficient geriatric assessment and subsequent triage of appropriately targeted at risk individuals to care management systems which promote functional health. Focusing health resources on the ambulatory care management of chronic disease is necessary to appropriately manage overall health of the frail elderly. Ambulatory chronic care case management is a fundamental and primary strategy for promoting the quality and reducing the costs of caring for the frail elderly.

The frail elderly are at risk for poor health care outcomes and adverse health events which may result in frequent ambulatory care visits, admission to a hospital or other institutions such as a nursing home. In the frail elderly, as in other populations, quality of care and cost of care are intimately linked. As a result of the common occurrence of adverse health events among the frail elderly, this population of geriatric patients accounts for the majority of health care costs generated by the elderly. For example, about 25% of the Medicare population generally accounts for 90% of the total costs. While the frail elderly, roughly defined as individuals over the age of 75 years, represent 13% of the total population over the age of 65 years in Medicare HMOs, they consume approximately 55% of costs in managed Medicare programs.

The Process Of Comprehensive, Multidisciplinary Geriatric Care

There are well-established, sequential steps in the process of geriatric assessment. Essentially, these include: 1) *high risk screening* to identify the frail elderly members at risk; 2) *geriatric assessment* to further evaluate these patients and 3) *effective and efficient triage* to comprehensive, multidisciplinary geriatric care management.

High risk screening may be performed using validated questionnaires which have demonstrated predictive validity for future health care utilization. These instruments may be performed either telephonically, in person, or through the mail. Generally, about 5-10% of members in a health plan or normally selected population representative of a normal population will be high risk. This information is useful in predicting geriatric case management needs.

A number of variables can be employed for high risk screening. Recent research in this area has investigated the predictive validity of these variables and incorporated them into scores to identify individuals who are at high risk for increased medical utilization. Presumably, increased medical utilization is a proxy for poor health outcomes and functional decline, although this has not been clearly established. Nevertheless, high risk screens have value in assisting in the identification of members who may benefit from geriatric assessment (screening followed by targeted geriatric assessment). In managed care, these high risk individuals are generally referred to geriatric case management. Brief questionnaires for high risk screening have been published.

After assessment and identification of high risk, frail elderly patients, implementation of recommended care plans is coordinated with the primary care physicians. Each high risk frail elderly patient is assigned to a multidisciplinary primary geriatric care team.

Geriatric care management protocols and clinical practice guidelines are made available to the team and the Primary Care Provider (PCP). These protocols include assessment and management strategies for common, specific geriatric problems (eg. falls, polypharmacy, urinary incontinence, dementia).

The protocols address the issue of standardization of care to reduce variability and costs through both medical management as well as systems management (eg. sole sourcing for rehabilitation, home health care and disease management programs).

After initial geriatric assessments have been performed by individual team members, team meetings are held to develop a multidisciplinary plan for ongoing geriatric care. Team members must be trained in the conduct of multidisciplinary team meetings. At the team meeting, a coordinated, multidisciplinary care plan is developed. The geriatric care team is responsible for implementation of the plan.

Figure 1. The Process of Geriatric Assessment in Traditional Ambulatory Care

PCP sees patient in initial medical visit

Patient is informally identified as a high risk patient or may receive a high risk screen during a regular visit

Proactive screening of a population is unusual in the private physician's practice, but may occur in large medical groups with this capability

A nurse may further assess the patient employing validated instruments

Team meeting typically difficult to arrange because of time pressures: however, nurse and physician may meet to discuss case. Generally, a social worker is not immediately available, but a referral may be made through a home health agency, community agency or a private social worker

Identification of needs and development of an initial care plan

Care plan is discussed with patient and caregiver

Care plan is implemented by team

Periodic review of care plan by physician

Geriatric Assessment in Managed Care

Success in the delivery of managed health care for the frail elderly depends on the ability of an organization to provide coordinated care through an *integrated geriatric care delivery system,* from the home, to the office, hospital, subacute care, nursing home, rehabilitation facility, daycare center. Operating within this system, *a multidisciplinary team with geriatric expertise* in several required disciplines must be able to effectively communicate and execute the geriatric team approach. An interdisciplinary team is required because of the multidisciplinary nature of the health problems suffered by the geriatric patient. The multidisciplinary geriatric team is essential in providing high quality, efficient geriatric care which ultimately reduces costs. We liken the geriatric system to the hardware of geriatrics, while the team is the software without which the system cannot run.

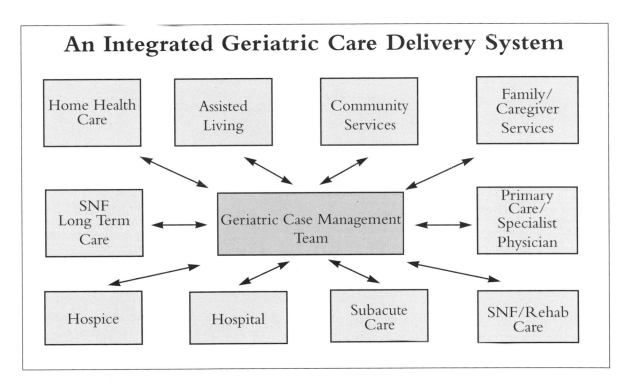

An Integrated Geriatric Care Delivery System

In managed care, there are a number of challenges to the implementation of geriatric assessment. Part of the challenge lies in the structure of the HMO itself. Staff models, such as Kaiser-Permanente, will have little difficulty implementing geriatric assessment programs, should they choose to do so, because the insurer and the provider are one and the same organization. However, the evolving dominant of model managed care in the U.S. is the group model or the independent practice association (IPA) model. In these latter systems, the insurer and the provider are separate organizations. In the IPA model, physicians remain in solo or small group practices with little organizational structure. This means that there are often few resources for programs such as high risk screening, geriatric assessment, geriatric case management, or multidisciplinary team care. In these settings, the health plan, or managed care organization, may represent the only organizational structure available for the development of geriatric care programs.

However, financial incentives and barriers, particularly capitation, ultimately play a crucial role in these relationships. If a provider group such as an IPA is fully capitated or has taken full risk for a population, they are fully responsible for the care of geriatric patients.

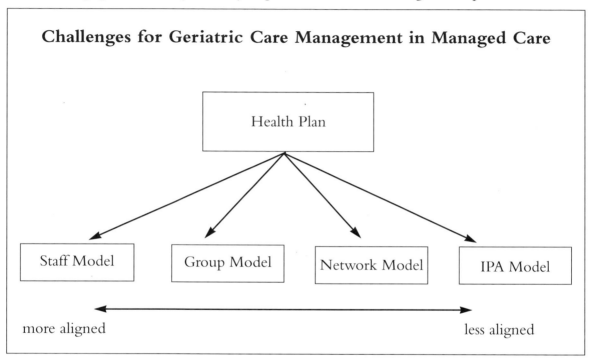

Challenges for Geriatric Care Management in Managed Care

Health Plan

Staff Model   Group Model   Network Model   IPA Model

more aligned   less aligned

For these groups, high risk screening, geriatric assessment, and geriatric case management makes both financial and clinical sense because it leads to cost-effective, high quality care. However, in the traditional fee-for-service Medicare health system, there are few equivalent financial incentives or opportunities for the development of such quality geriatric programs.

There are many methods for conducting geriatric assessment in the managed care setting. These are dependent on the setting and structure of the managed care plan. Generally, the conduct of geriatric assessment is performed as a form of specialized case management. In a fully capitated program, case management may be done by the provider group. However, in shared risk programs, case management may be based in the health plan. Regardless of the financial and clinical arrangements in the managed care setting, geriatric case managers often conduct the initial assessment. The geriatric assessment is then discussed with the PCP, preferably after the PCP has seen the patient for an initial visit. This may occur in person or telephonically. Obviously, the quality of the assessment process is more clinically effective when conducted with all team members together in the same room, but this is not always desirable or possible. For example, some health plans may provide coverage to very large geographic regions. The conference (either telephonic or in person) between the geriatric case manager and the PCP has several purposes: 1) the GNP, as a representative of the health plan, obtains accurate medical information from the PCP; 2) the PCP obtains information on the multiple geriatric health problems of the patient, and the suggested geriatric care plans to address these problems; 3) the geriatric case manager will also have the opportunity to explain to the PCP the clinical resources available to the PCP to assist in their care of the complex needs of the frail elderly. The geriatric case manager may also have the opportunity to provide educational materials and advice to the PCP in geriatric care in a non-threatening manner through the development of a personal therapeutic rapport with the PCP. The geriatric case manager may need to conduct outreach visits to skilled nursing facilities, convalescent homes, and individual seniors homes for the express purpose of chronic disease assessment beyond the capabilities of a home nursing or other home health agency visit.

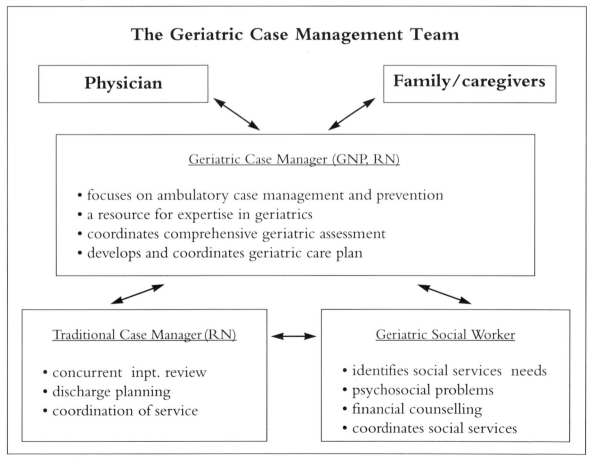

In most health systems, there is also a need for providers, including physicians, nurses, social workers and others, with geriatric expertise. This has a strong basis in the knowledge and practice of geriatrics. There is a significant body of knowledge in geriatrics which is not generally known by traditional providers. There are also marked differences in practice styles between geriatric care providers and traditional providers. Geriatric care generally requires a focus on the management of multiple, chronic, generally incurable and progressive diseases; seeking the multifactorial causes of health problems with a goal towards finding reversibility; an emphasis on the promotion of functional health; the provision of humane, appropriate care which dispels "ageism"; the ability to work effectively with a multidiscplinary team; and knowledge of the long term care chronic disease management systems necessary to implement geriatric care. Developing this expertise in health systems is an important challenge that is frequently difficult to meet because of a lack of commitment by the organization, a lack of personnel with geriatric expertise, and the perception that the frail elderly are just like everyone else. This attitude has proven to be a fatal mistake in many Medicare managed care programs.

Multidisciplinary geriatric care programs must offer primary care physicians "added value" service by providing the resources and expertise they need to manage the complex health care needs of the frail elderly. In most physician offices, there is a lack of expertise and resources in clinical geriatric care management needed to effectively manage high risk patients. For example, few solo practitioners in IPAs or group practices have immediate access to a social worker. To motivate the primary care practitioner to participate in geriatric case management programs, the "added value" of the program to the practitioner must be fairly obvious and immediate and must actually reduce the burden of caring for this complex population by providing the additional resources (ie. the multidisiciplinary team and the necessary systems and resources) to complement and supplement the traditional primary care physician's capacity to meet the complex, multidisciplinary needs of the frail elderly.

In an era of cost containment and managed care, the added expenditure for geriatric care teams is well justified. Case management programs have been previously demonstrated to be cost-effective. As a specialized form of case management, geriatric case management targets the frail elderly. As these patients may have very high cost expenditures, prevention of even one or two hospitalizations during the course of a year can often pay the salary of a geriatric case manager and a geriatric social worker. In terms of staffing, in a normally selected Medicare population of approximately 10,000 patients with approximately 5% high risk members requiring geriatric assessment and geriatric care management, approximately 500 patients would require geriatric case management. This would reasonably represent an initial caseload for approximately 2-3 case managers, depending on the availability of financial resources and the urgency with which these patients are needed to be entered into the geriatric case management program.

Figure 2. The Process of Geriatric Assessment in Managed Care

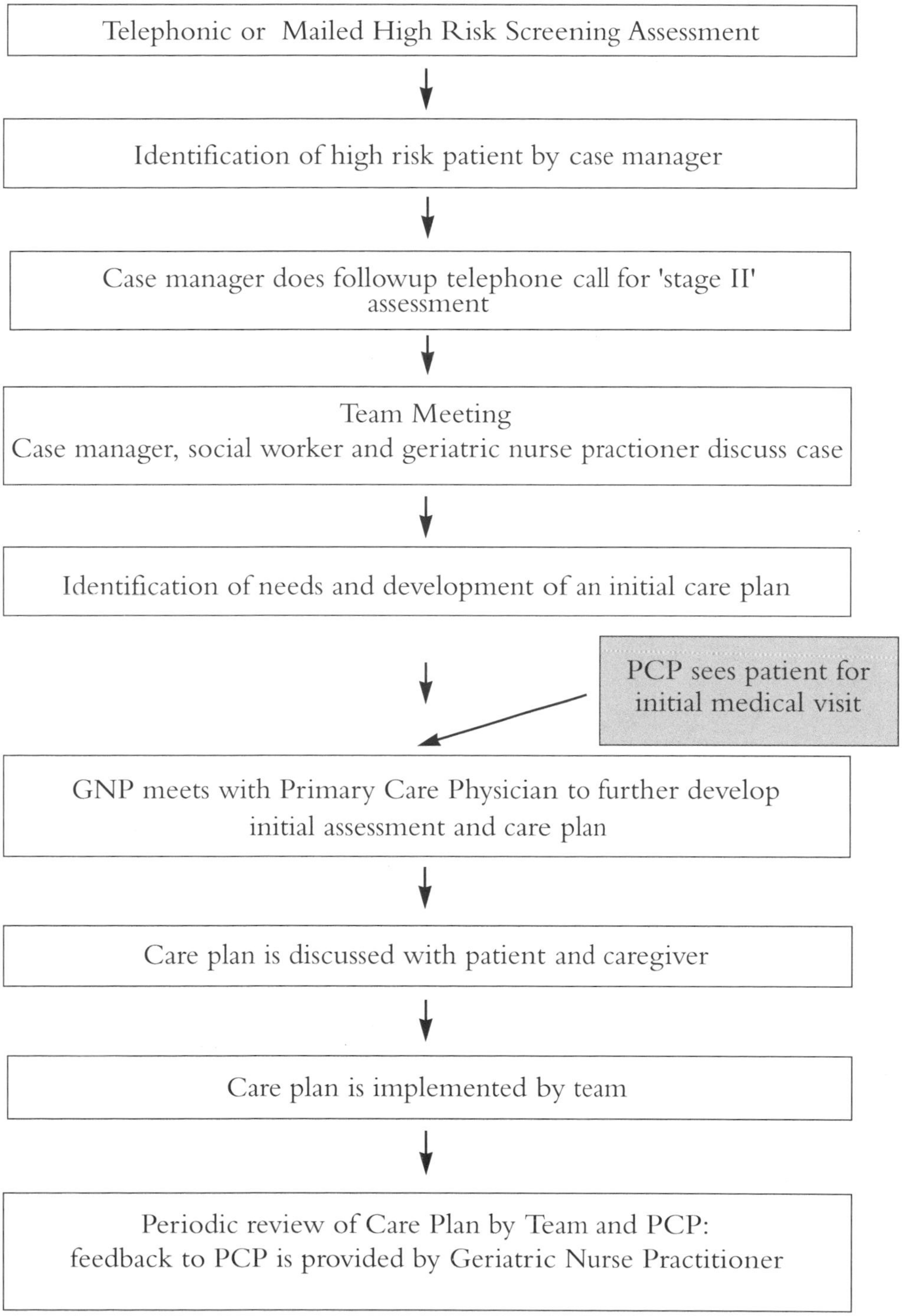

Telephonic or Mailed High Risk Screening Assessment

↓

Identification of high risk patient by case manager

↓

Case manager does followup telephone call for 'stage II' assessment

↓

Team Meeting
Case manager, social worker and geriatric nurse practioner discuss case

↓

Identification of needs and development of an initial care plan

↓

PCP sees patient for initial medical visit

GNP meets with Primary Care Physician to further develop initial assessment and care plan

↓

Care plan is discussed with patient and caregiver

↓

Care plan is implemented by team

↓

Periodic review of Care Plan by Team and PCP:
feedback to PCP is provided by Geriatric Nurse Practitioner

HIGH RISK SCREENING INSTRUMENT -- P_{ra}
(Probability of Repeated Admissions).

This instrument has demonstrated predictive validity to identify individuals most at risk for high utilization of health care resources. The P_{ra} is administered by direct mailing, telephonic or person-to-person interview. Screening data are used to compute a risk score for each individual. Thresholds must be established that divide these scores into risk categories, such as low, moderate and high. Historically, persons with P_{ra} scores of 0.5 or greater have twice the hospital days and costs of those with scores below 0.5. About 7% of the general elderly population and 18% of Medicaid elderly population have risk scores of 0.5 or higher.

In general would you say your health is:

Excellent   Very Good   Good   Fair   Poor

In the previous 12 months have you stayed overnight as a patient in a hospital?

Not at all   1 time   2-3 times   More than 3 times

In the previous 12 months how many times did you visit a physician or clinic?

Not at all   1 time   2-3 times   4-6 times   More than 6 times

In the previous 12 months did you have diabetes?   Yes   No

Have you ever had: Coronary Artery Disease?   Yes   No
Angina Pectoris?   Yes   No
A Myocardial Infarction?   Yes   No

Your sex?   **Male**   **Female**

Is there is a friend, relative or neighbor who would take care of you for a few days, if necessary   Yes   No

Your date of birth?   Month   Date   Year

P_{ra} Scoring Formula

$$P_{ra} = \frac{e^{BX}}{1 + e^{BX}}$$

$$BX = -1.802 + .327X_1 + .340X_2 + .552X_3 + .770X_4 + .390X_5 = .545X_6$$
$$+ .318X_7 - .738X_8 + .255X_9 + .327X_{10} + .559x_{11} + .257X_{12} + .319X_{13}$$

Predictor variables: 0 = absent   1 = present

X_1	very good general health
X_2	good general health
X_3	fair general health
X_4	poor general health
X_5	coronary heart disease
X_6	hospital admissions in the last year
X_7	> 6 physicians visits in past year
X_8	no informal caregivers available
X_9	age 75-79 years
X_{10}	age 80-84 years
X_{11}	age 85+ years
X_{12}	male sex
X_{13}	diabetes in past year

Adapted from:

Pacala, J.T., Boult, C., Reed, R.L., Aliberti, E. Predictive validity of the P_{ra} instrument among older recipients of managed care. *J. Amer. Geriatr. Soc.* 1997 **45**: 614-617.

Guidelines for Referral to the Geriatric Team for Geriatric Assessment:

The primary care physician should have adequate knowledge in geriatric medicine necessary for providing quality health care of the elderly. Such knowledge includes, but is not limited to:

1. Understanding general principles of geriatrics and gerontology, including

   • the heterogeneity of the elderly (the continuum from the well elderly to the frail elderly);

   • normal human aging and its clinical significance, such as age-related changes in organ function and laboratory tests;

   • unique aspects of the history, physical exam and diagnosis in the elderly including the altered presentation of disease and the multifactorial nature of illness;

   • appropriate medication prescribing practices in the elderly, goals of geriatric care (caring not curing, a focus on maintenance of functional independence and quality of life).

2. The primary care physician should have clinical knowledge in specific areas of geriatric medicine necessary for quality primary care of the elderly, including:

   • unique aspects of preventive medicine in both the young-old and the old-old (for example, appropriate use of exercise, immunizations, cancer screening, prevention of falls).

   • diagnosis, management and treatment of diseases and geriatric syndromes common in the frail elderly, including but not limited to: dementia, depression, delirium, falls, functional decline, immobility, and rehabilitation; malnutrition, pressure sores, polypharmacy, sensory impairments (hearing and vision loss), sleep disorders, urinary and fecal incontinence. When further specialized cognitive services, testing or surgical care is required for diagnosis, management or treatment, referral to an appropriate specialist for the above problems, including the geriatrician, is indicated.

   • the clinical significance of social factors, such as caregiver stress and social isolation, affecting health in the elderly.

   • knowledge of ethics as it pertains to decision making and clinical care in the elderly, including advanced directives.

• knowledge of the basic principles and practice of long term care, hospice and palliative care, including pain management.

3. The primary care physician should specifically refer patients to a geriatrician for the following reasons:

• diagnosis, management and treatment of frail elderly patients with complex, multi-disciplinary (medical, functional and psychosocial) health problems requiring a comprehensive geriatric assessment by the geriatrician and an interdisciplinary geriatric team in order to discover reversible causes of illness and decline, promote functional independence and quality of life and develop a comprehensive, long term care plan for the primary care physician.

• patients with diagnoses or geriatric syndromes (as briefly described above) for whom consultation with an expert geriatrician may be of benefit for diagnosis, management or treatment.

• patients requiring long term care, such as care in a skilled nursing home or home care, where the geriatrician, by virtue of their practice patterns and their expertise in these settings, provides efficient access and/or availability and promotes quality care in settings not familiar to the primary care physician.

GERIATRIC ASSESSMENT IN THE ACUTE CARE SETTING

Acute care geriatric services have been an integral part of acute hospital care throughout the world for more than twenty years. Acute geriatric inpatient units represent an organizational approach to the complex, interdisciplinary problems of hospitalized frail elderly patients whose health care needs often extend beyond the treatment of a single acute medical illness. These units also serve as model sites to foster the development of innovative methods of care for frail elderly patients in the hospital setting, and as a teaching site for geriatrics. Although relatively new to hospitals in the United States, incorporation of geriatric care into the acute care setting has occured progressively during the past twenty years. This has occured through the development of inpatient acute care geriatric units and geriatric consultation services.

Acute geriatric care units for the hospitalized frail elderly specialize in the complex, unique, and interdisciplinary aspects of illness in the aged. Since these patients often have multiple chronic illnesses, the goal of geriatric care is the restoration and maintenance of function essential to the preservation of a reasonable quality of life. Acute geriatric care involves the close cooperation of patients, family members and other caregivers with the geriatric team to consider the difficult decisions affecting the treatment of acute illness in the frail elderly patient.

Comprehensive geriatric assessment is an essential component of geriatric care in the acute setting, to insure that all of the frail elderly patient's complex health care needs are met during their hospital stay, particularly for frail elderly patients with complex health care problems in whom outpatient assessment may be difficult or impossible. Comprehensive geriatric assessment in the acute setting is accomplished through the multidisciplinary team approach and the use of an organized, efficient set of "instruments" and procedures to insure that the assessment process does not unduly prolong hospital length of stay.

The multidisciplinary team is the foundation of specialized acute geriatric care in the acute geriatric care unit. Geriatricians and primary care providers focus on the unique problems of the frail elderly and the very old, such as the diagnostic evaluation of cognitive impairment, falls and other problems. Geriatric nursing provides expert specialized management and treatment of decubiti, incontinence, feeding disorders and other skilled nursing problems. Psychosocial problems are managed by a geriatric social worker who provides counselling to patients and caregivers, and assists in obtaining services to ensure efficient and appropriate discharge placement and posthospitalization care. Finally, geriatric consultant specialists in neurology, nutrition, pharmacology, psychiatry, psychology and rehabilitation are an integral part of the acute geriatric care team.

The performance of geriatric assessment in the acute care setting must be an efficient and comprehensive process which does not significantly prolong hospital length of stay. The additional presence of a geographically-based interdisciplinary team and the use of this handbook or similar organizational devices greatly facilitates this process. The geriatric assessment must be performed in a coordinated, efficient fashion in conjunction with primary medical care during the course of the patient's acute illness and does not result in extended stays. This is not only important under Medicare Prospective Payment, but becomes particularly important in an era of managed care.

Some frail patients may require admission to the acute geriatric unit for geriatric assessment even though they do not have traditional diagnoses or problems that would usually provide them access to hospital acute care beds under traditional Medicare Prospective Payment in the United States or even other countries. However, many Diagnosis Related Groups (DRGs) of the Medicare Prospective Payment System are applicable to our frail elderly patient population and can be employed for admitting patients to the acute geriatric unit who are progressively deteriorating and require comprehensive geriatric assessment. In addition to the usual acute care diagnoses, a number of DRG diagnoses are applicable to the frail population that are not commonly employed, such as Alzheimer's disease or senile dementia (DRG category #12 or #430); decubiti (DRG category #271); urinary incontinence (DRG category # 325); sleep disorders (DRG category #432); cachexia, malnutrition, or weight loss (DRG category #463 or 297). However, diagnosis alone is not the sole criterion for approval of admission. Each DRG has criteria for acute care which must be demonstrated, both on admission and in a retrospective review that "something was done" in the hospital which justified hospitalization.

An important concept regarding hospitalization of patients for geriatric assessment is that of multiple diagnoses or problems in frail elderly patients for whom the "sum" is greater than the "parts". That is, in an individual patient, while no single diagnosis alone might justify an admission, a multitude of diagnoses might equal an "acute" admission. For example, for some frail complex patients, numerous clinic visits over the course of several months might be required to complete an evaluation for multiple medical problems, during which time a frail elderly patient might progressively deteriorate as a result of unresolved problems. Such patients might benefit from a short term hospitalization with an assessment and treatment which might accomplish the same objectives during the course of a few days. The benefit of hospitalization might be to prevent morbidity from problems which would be otherwise unresolved and progressive for long periods, as well as a reduction in the stress of numerous transfers to and from home and long waiting periods sitting in ambulatory offices. Although there are obvious risks associated with hospitalization, these might be outweighed by the benefits of relatively quick and comprehensive resolution of complex problems. Whether such strategies can be demonstrated to be cost-effective, particularly in a managed care environment remains to be seen. In managed care, a variety of alternate strategies might be available to avert a costly, and potentially dangerous, inpatient stay. Nevertheless, even in managed care there are likely situations when inpatient geriatric assessment is justified and cost-effective.

In all cases, documentation in the hospital chart of the need for hospitalization is essential in obtaining approval for payment from Medicare or managed care payers. Narratives explaining exactly why hospitalization is necessary in a frail patient, if reasonable, are extremely valuable in justifying admissions and continued stays.

The Process of Geriatric Assessment in the Acute Care Setting

This book can be used as a guide for comprehensive geriatric assessment of patients in the acute setting. Most of the assessments are relevant and applicable to a frail, hospitalized geriatric population and address problems commonly encountered in this setting. The admission geriatric assessment should include an admission history and physical examination. The process of comprehensive geriatric assessment is facilitated and organized by the "Screening Questionnaire" to identify patients needing specific assessments. The admission comprehensive geriatric assessment should be completed within 48 hours of admission, and summarized by a **"Geriatric Assessment"admission note** in the patient's medical record. Problems identified on admission assessment can be noted on the "Checklist," which is designed as a summary and progress sheet. Progress notes concerning the results of the geriatric assessment process should also be included in the medical record. The results of the assessment process should be discussed with the multidisciplinary staff and caregivers.

In the academic setting, this process also provides an opportunity for teaching geriatric assessment to medical students, housestaff, geriatric fellows, nurses, social workers and other providers. In academic programs, or in nonacademic programs with geriatric services, often the geriatric assessment is done by a Fellow, or by a geriatrician as part of a consultation service. In hospitals without geriatric units but with a geriatrician or geriatric programs, geriatric assessments are often done throughout the hospital as part of a geriatric consultation service.

ADMISSION CRITERIA: Acute Care Geriatric Units

Acute geriatric care units provide intensive, interdisciplinary, comprehensive geriatric assessment and geriatric specialty care for the frail elderly.

I. Inclusion criteria: Frail elderly patients

a) Over the age of 65 years; generally over 75 years old

b) Meet Medicare Prospective Payment "guidelines" for **acute care**

c) **Complex, multidisciplinary health care problems,** multiple medical co-morbidities, nursing and social problems requiring inpatient comprehensive geriatric assessment

d) Medically ill patients with **Specialty Problems in Geriatric Medicine**. A few examples are:

- cognitive and affective disorders
- falls, immobility and gait disorders
- urinary and fecal incontinence
- malnutrition and feeding disorders
- complications of polypharmacy
- pressure sores
- sensory impairments
- sleep disorders
- elder abuse associated with medical co-morbidities

e) Patients should have the **POTENTIAL TO BENEFIT** from intensive, inpatient geriatric assessment, rehabilitation, management and treatment services to restore function.

II. Exclusion criteria: Acute geriatric care units are NOT:

1) a hospice or a palliative care unit; in addition, patients with severe cognitive impairment are generally excluded, as they will not maximally benefit from acute geriatric care services (although these patients are occasionally admitted for specialized geriatric care);

2) a "geriatric ICU"; patients requiring intensive care should be transferred to the Intensive Care Unit.

3) an alternate level of care unit for elderly patients solely requiring or awaiting nursing home placement or home care services.

ASSESSMENT SCREENING QUESTIONNAIRE

This is a brief questionnaire which can be employed by the practitioner to determine specific areas of need in individuals who have already been identified as high risk (see above). The questionnaire is an attempt to organize the process of initiating a comprehensive geriatric assessment in a high risk individual by identifying the primary components of geriatric assessment which will require further assessment. To do this, the questionnaire employs brief, relevant questions in each area of assessment. Some of the questions are derived from items that have been validated. The questionnaire should not replace the clinicians' history, physical examination and clinical judgement as to which areas of geriatric assessment should be investigated further. The instrument should simply be considered a device for focusing and prioritizing efforts in patients with complex, multidisciplinary needs, and insuring that the process of assessment is comprehensive. For each question circle the appropriate letter. If the response to an item is Yes, then that area should be further assessed using the provided tools.

A. ALCOHOL ABUSE

Y N   Does the patient or caregiver give a history of use of alcohol on a regular basis?

B. CAREGIVER STRESS

Y N   Does the caregiver feel overwhelmed in caring for the patient?

Y N   Have the caregivers or geriatric team noted problems with the quality of care provided to the patient?

C. COGNITIVE IMPAIRMENT

Y N   Does the patient or the caregiver complain of problems with the patient's memory?

Y N   Ask the patient to repeat three items (eg. boat, chair, dog). Can the patient NOT recall these items after 3 minutes? If the patient cannot recall three items, perform the MiniMental Status examination.

D. DEPRESSION

Y N   Does the patient often feel sad or depressed?

Y N   Has the patient exhibited a recent change in personality, with more anxiety, aggressive behavior, or apathy?

E. ELDER ABUSE AND NEGLECT

Y N   Is there a suspicion of abuse or neglect by history or on physical examination?

Y N   Is there a potential for the patient to be placed in an environment that may put them at risk for abuse or neglect?

F. FALLS ASSESSMENT
Y N   Does the patient have a history of falls?

Y N   Does the patient report gait abnormalities?

G. FUNCTIONAL ASSESSMENT
Y N   Does the patient require supervision or assistance with shopping, household chores such as cooking, laundry, cleaning or basic activities such as dressing, bathing, or toileting?

H. HEALTH MAINTENANCE
Y N   Has the patient NOT had adequate health maintenance measures in the past?

Y N   Does the patient wish to pursue health maintenance measures?

I. HEARING IMPAIRMENT
Y N   Does the patient exhibit evidence of poor hearing?

Y N   Does the patient or caregiver complain of a deterioration in patient's hearing status?

J. IMMUNOCOMPETENCE
Y N   Does the patient suffer from recurrent infections?

Y N   Is the patient NOT current on all their immunizations?

K. INCONTINENCE: FECAL
Y N   Does the patient or caregiver complain of problems with incontinence?

Y N   Does the nursing record reveal episodes of incontinence?

L. INCONTINENCE: URINARY
Y N   Has the patient been incontinent of urine during the past six months?

M. INSTITUTIONALIZATION RISK
Y N   Did social factors play an important role in the admission of this patient?

Y N   Has the patient's status deteriorated such that institutionalization should be considered?

N. NUTRITIONAL ASSESSMENT
Y N   Has the patient lost more than 10 pounds over the past six months without trying to do so?

Y N   Is the patient below 90% of ideal body weight or do they have an albumin of <3.5?

O. ORAL AND DENTAL ASSESSMENT
Y N   Has the patient NOT been to the dentist within the past year?

Y N   Does the patient complain of or are there on physical examination dental problems?

P. OSTEOPOROSIS
Y N   Has the patient had fractures of the spine, distal forearm, or proximal femur, or do they have evidence of osteopenia on Xray?

Y N   Is the patient at risk for the development of osteoporosis?

Q. PALLIATIVE CARE PLANNING
Y N   Does the patient NOT have an advanced directive?

Y N   Is the patient suffering a terminal or preterminal illness?

R. POLYPHARMACY
Y N   Does the patient take more than five medications?

Y N   Has the patient's medication regimen NOT been reviewed for appropriateness and compliance problems?

S. PREOPERATIVE ASSESSMENT
Y N   To be completed on all patients scheduled for a surgical procedure

T. PRESSURE ULCERS
Y N   Has the patient had any problems with skin integrity?

Y N   Does the Nursing Staff's assessment indicate risk for decubitus formation?

U. REHABILITATION
Y N   Have areas been identified in the patient's functional assessment that may benefit from an assessment by a physiatrist?

Y N   Is the patient in need of assistive devices, reconditioning, or assessment because of mobility problems?

V. SLEEP DISORDER
Y N   Does the patient or caregiver complain of problems with sleeping?

Y N   Has an altered sleep pattern been exhibited by the patient?

W. VISUAL IMPAIRMENT
Y N   Does the patient have difficulty driving, watching television or reading, or performing other daily activities because of vision problems?

Y N   Has the patient or caregiver noted a decline in vision?

Completed by _____

ASSESSMENT TOOL CHECKLIST

This tool assists the practioner in documenting and tracking to completion the elements of geriatric assessment that are needed and will be performed.

Functional Assessment			
Functional Assessment			
Rehabilitation			
Medical Assessment			
Advanced directives			
Alcohol abuse			
Falls assessment			
Health maintenance			
Immunocompetence			
Incontinence: Fecal			
Incontinence: Urinary			
Nutritional health			
Oral and dental health			
Osteoporosis			
Polypharmacy			
Pre-opearitive assessment			
Pressure ulcers			
Sensory impairment: Hearing			
Sensory impairment: Vision			
Sleep disorders			
Affective Cognitive Assessment			
Affective disorders			
Cognitive impairment			
Social Assessment			
Caregiver stress			
Elder abuse and negelct			
Institutionalization risk			

Completed by: _____

PART II. COMPREHENSIVE GERIATRIC ASSESSMENT

FUNCTIONAL ASSESSMENT

FUNCTIONAL ASSESSMENT OF THE OLDER ADULT

Significance of Impaired Function in Older Adults

The ability to function independently is determined by an individual's capability to complete every day activities. Measurements of ability to complete **instrumental activities of daily living** (shopping, preparing meals, administering medications to self, managing finances, utilizing transportation, performing housekeeping skills and executing use of telephone) are included in a functional assessment. The second component of a functional assessment is measurement of ability for completion of **activities of daily living** (bathing, dressing, feeding self, toiletting, maintaining continence and transferring). Advanced activities of daily living include the ability to participate in social and/or occupational activities.

Increasing age and the presence of chronic health conditions impact on the older adults ability to successfully complete these activities independently. As many as 40% of older adults have some limitations in their ability to complete instrumental activities of daily living and/or activities of daily living. If attention is not paid to functional decline, the older adult may become progressively more dependent. This increased dependency leads to poor quality of life, frequent hospitalizations and/or need for more intensive long term care. Finally low functional ability is a strong predictor of mortality in older adults.

Etiology

In addition to changes associated with increasing age, such as decreased vision and declining muscle strength, several disease states contribute to functional decline in the older adult, including, muscloskeletal conditions (osteoarthritis, osteoporosis), diabetes, degenerative neurological diseases e.g. dementia, Parkinson's disease, cerebrovascular disease, malnutrition and depression.

Diagnosis

Medical History

An open ended question such as "Tell me how you spend your day" will elicit much information about functional ability. Thereafter, more direct questions generate precise and quantitative responses to the specific tasks in question. In the event that the individual is not a reliable historian due to dementia, delirium or denial, it will be important to include a family member and/or informal caregiver in this interview process.

Physical exam

Attention to the individual's personal appearance and grooming will provide information regarding ability for completion of activities of daily living. The clinician should observe cleanliness and appropriateness of clothing, condition of hair and skin as well as dental hygiene. Specific activities to focus on include individual's ability at dressing and undressing (e.g. tying shoe laces, buttoning shirt, etc.) and ease of transfer from chair to upright position. A full neurologic and muscloskeletal evaluation with attention to muscle strength, range of motion and presence of weakness is helpful. Testing to assess cognitive function and presence of depression is appropriate if such mental problems are thought to contribute to functional decline.

Laboratory Testing

Based on reported history and physical findings, specific diagnostic tests help to determine etiology for functional decline in the older adult. These may include laboratory studies such as thyroid function testing, vitamin B12 and folate levels, Complete Blood Count and Chemistries.

Treatment and Management

Assessment of an older adult's functional capacity and implementation of management strategies to address the individual's needs are essential to maximize physical, psychological and social well being. The recognition of undiagnosed and treatable conditions which contribute to functional decline can be determined by the completion of an appropriate evaluation.

In addition to treating any underlying conditions, the utilization of a multidisciplinary approach is critical in addressing issues related to functional impairment in older adults.

Social services can refer patients to community agencies to assist in execution of IADL's and ADL's for the older adult. These resources may include homemaker/home health aid services, medical adult day care, respite care and mobile meals. Assessment of family dynamics with emphasis on family member/caregiver burden and potential for elder neglect or abuse will also be accomplished. Finally, the social worker can provide information regarding availability of alternative living arrangements, such as assisted living and life care facilities.

An occupational therapist can perform a home safety evaluation with possible recommendations for adaptive devices, such as grab bars in bathroom, raised toilet seat and shower seat.

Strengthening and conditioning exercises, gait training and use of assistive devices for ambulation will be accomplished through a referral for physical therapy.

If visual problems are contributing to functional impairment, an ophthalmology consult and/or referral for low vision aids is appropriate.

Discussion to facilitate older adult's and family member's understanding of importance of advanced directives is essential. The completion of an advanced medical directive allows the frail older adult to give instructions about future medical care needs. Health care professionals and family members are then guided by these instructions should the individual no longer be able to make decisions.

Summary

Maintaining functional independence and quality of life are the primary goals of geriatric care. Performing a functional assessment is crucial to evaluate the geriatric patient, identifying reversal causes of functional decline, preventing further decline and maximizing independence. Functional assessments are necessary for older adults in all clinical settings. Based on the degree of functional impairment and the presence of comorbidity, follow-up re-evaluations should be completed periodically.

FUNCTIONAL ASSESSMENT

INSTRUMENTAL ACTIVITIES OF DAILY LIVING

The purpose of this instrument is to evaluate the functional ability of elderly persons on different levels of competence, in particular, autonomy in ambulatory physical and "instrumental" activities of daily living.

A. ABILITY TO USE TELEPHONE

1	1.	Operates telephone on own initiative
1	2.	Dials a few well-known numbers
1	3.	Answers telephone but does not dial
0	4.	Does not use telephone at all

B. SHOPPING

1	1.	Takes care of all shopping needs independently
0	2.	Shops independently for small purchases
0	3.	Needs to be accompanied on any shopping trip
0	4.	Completely unable to shop

C. FOOD PREPARATION

1	1.	Plans, prepares, and serves adequate meals independently
0	2.	Prepares adequate meals if supplied with ingredients
0	3.	Heats, serves and prepares meals, or prepares meals, but does not maintain adequate diet
0	4.	Needs to have meals prepared and served

D. HOUSEKEEPING

1	1.	Maintains house alone or with occasional assistance
1	2.	Performs light daily tasks such as dishwashing or bedmaking
1	3.	Performs light daily tasks but cannot maintain acceptable level of cleanliness
1	4.	Needs help with all home maintenance tasks
0	5.	Does not participate in any housekeeping tasks

E. LAUNDRY

1	1.	Does personal laundry completely
1	2.	Launders small items by self
0	3.	All laundry must be done by others

F. MODE OF TRANSPORTATION

1	1.	Travels independently
1	2.	Arranges own travel via taxi, but does not use other modes of transportation
1	3.	Travels on public transportation when accompanied by others
1	4.	Travel limited to full assistance by others
0	5.	Does not travel at all

G. RESPONSIBILITY FOR MEDICATIONS

1	1.	Is able to take medications in correct dosages at correct time
0	2.	Takes medications if they are prepared in advance in correct dosages
0	3.	Is not capable of dispensing own medications

H. ABILITY TO HANDLE FINANCES

1	1.	Manages financial matters independently
1	2.	Manages day-to-day purchases but needs help with banking, major purchases, etc.
0	3.	Incapable of handling money, etc.

_____

TOTAL

(For each item the score can only be 1 or 0.)

Completed by _____

Adapted from: Lawton., M.P. and Brody, E.M. Assessment of older people: self-maintaining and instrumental activities of daily living. *Gerontologist* 1969 **9**: 179–186

FUNCTIONAL ASSESSMENT

ACTIVITIES OF DAILY LIVING

This tool is designed to serve as a measure of objective evaluation of activities of daily living.

CIRCLE THE APPROPRIATE SCORE FOR EACH ITEM

1. BATHING – either sponge bath or shower
   - 0 – without assistance
   - 1 – needs help getting in or out of the tub, or special attachments, or in bathing one part of the body
   - 2 – unable to bathe self or needs assistance with bathing more than one part of the body

2. DRESSING – includes choosing and obtaining clothing
   - 0 – without help
   - 1 – needs assistance (e.g. with tying shoes)
   - 2 – unable to dress and undress self and requires assistance

3. TOILETING – going to toilet, cleaning self, and changing clothes
   - 0 – without assistance. May use bedside commode or bedpan at night, but is able to empty the receptacle in the morning
   - 1 – needs assistance in either getting to the bathroom, cleaning self after elimination, arranging clothes, or returning from the bathroom
   - 2 – unable to go to bathroom for elimination

4. TRANSFER – can get in and out of bed and on and off chair
   - 0 – without assistance except for cane or walker
   - 1 – needs some assistance
   - 2 – unable to get out of bed

5. CONTINENCE – both urine and bowel function completely by self
   - 0 – able to control bowel and urine function by self
   - 1 – has occasional "accidents"
   - 2 – needs supervision, has catheter, or is incontinent

6. FEEDING
   - 0 – feeds self without assistance
   - 1 – feeds self but needs assistance with cutting meat, buttering bread, etc.
   - 2 – needs assistance in feeding or is being fed by IV or enteral feedings

FUNCTIONAL ASSESSMENT

ACTIVITIES OF DAILY LIVING

Scoring:

A - independent in all functions
B - independent in all but one function
C - independent in all but bathing and one additional function
D - independent in all but bathing, dressing and one additional function
E - independent in all but bathing, dressing, toileting, and one additional function
F - independent in all but bathing, dressing, toileting, transferring and one additional function
G - dependent in all functions

SCORE _____   Completed by _____

Adapted from: Katz, S. et al. Studies of illness in the aged: The index of ADL; a standardized measure of biological and psychosocial function. *J. Amer. Med. Assoc.* 1963 **185**: 914-919.

REHABILITATION ASSESSMENT

The purpose of this tool is to identify those patients who may benefit from a rehabilitation program or the services of the rehabilitation department. In general, Rehabilitation Medicine should be consulted when any of the following problems are recognized:

Y	N	1.	The patient is deconditioned due to chronic medical conditions
Y	N	2.	The patient has become deconditioned due to recent surgery or other acute illness
Y	N	3.	The patient suffers from muscular weakness due to any medical condition
Y	N	4.	The patient has experienced a recent cerebrovascular accident
Y	N	5.	The patient is either at risk for the development of limb contractures or has contractures that may benefit from range of motion exercises or joint preservation techniques.
Y	N	6.	The patient has a gait disorder that may benefit from therapy
Y	N	7.	The patient has a disorder of balance that impairs the completion of daily activities
Y	N	8.	The patient has a need for assistive devices to enable the completion of daily activities
Y	N	9.	The patient's mobility problem requires prescription of specific equipment (i.e. wheelchairs, canes, prostheses)
Y	N	10.	The patient requires or may benefit from modalities other than medicines for the treatment of various arthritides, chronic pain syndromes, etc.
Y	N	11.	The patient is S/P limb amputation and requires stump training and/or fitting of prostheses
Y	N	12.	The patient requires training in transfers, stair climbing, or the negotiation of other obstacles
Y	N	13.	The patient has identified deficits in ADL's and IADL's.
Y	N	14.	The patient has sensory/perceptual deficits and may benefit from environmental modification.
Y	N	15.	The patient is aphasic, needs speech retraining, needs cognitive retraining, needs evaluation for a swallowing disorder, or could otherwise benefit from the services of a speech therapist.

NOTE: In order to benefit from consultations for the majority of the above problems, the patient must have the mental status sufficient to follow at least two-step commands and to retain instructions.

Completed by _____

GERIATRIC MEDICINE ASSESSMENT

ALCOHOL ABUSE

ASSESSING ALCOHOL MISUSE IN OLDER ADULTS

Significance of Problem

Although alcohol misuse is underreported and underdiagnosed, its prevalence among the elderly is estimated at about two to ten percent. Alcohol misuse is more common in older men than women.

Older adults are more sensitive to effects of alcohol because of their decreased lean body mass and total body water, comorbidities and interactions with concurrent medications. Alcohol use in the elderly aggravates existing medical conditions such as hypertension, diabetes, malnutrition, gout and dementia. Other consequences of alcohol use in the elderly include loss of functional abilities, falls, altered drug metabolism, altered mental status, urinary incontinence, Wernicke-Korsakoffi syndrome, cirrhosis and atrophic gastritis. Acute care hospitalization and admission to nursing home are common as a result of alcohol related problems among the elderly.

Alcohol use has significant psychological impact on the older adult as well as producing social isolation, self neglect and altered family relationships.

Etiology

Factors which place an older adult at risk for alcohol misuse include:

- genetic predisposition
- male gender
- insomnia
- personal losses
- depression
- chronic physical conditions
- chronic pain
- anxiety

Diagnosis

Medical History

Ask specific questions in a non-judgemental manner about type and frequency of alcohol consumption, quantities and setting in which drinking occurs. A family member should be utilized if the patient is a poor historian. Obtain a detailed medication history including over-the-counter drug use. Typical dietary intake, functional abilities, history of gastrointestinal complaints and cognitive impairment are also relevant. Finally, obtain a detailed medical history.

Physical Exam

Attention should be paid to overall physical appearance, personal hygiene and skin condition. Test for liver enlargement during abdominal exam. A neurologic exam should include assessment of gait, coordination and peripheral neuropathy. Mental status exam and depression testing are important components of the assessment process.

Laboratory Testing

Relevant laboratory studies include blood chemistries, Complete Blood Count, liver function tests, alkaline phosphatase and stool for guiac.

Treatment and Management

Treatment options will be based on the severity of alcohol misuse. Hospitalization for detoxification may be necessary. Underlying conditions, such as depression and malnutrition, and sequelae to alcohol use will require treatment interventions. Nonpharmaceutical interventions to relieve insomnia and anxiety should be introduced where appropriate.

In most cases, regardless of the clinical setting, a multidisciplinary approach to care will be most effective for long term therapy. An alcohol or psychiatric counselor will provide psychotherapy. Social service referral will introduce interventions, such as senior center participation to decrease social isolation. Nutritional counseling may be helpful.

Patient and family education is essential. This learning process should include consequence of alcohol, stress reduction strategies and benefits of participation in self help groups such as Alcoholics Anonymous and Al-anon.

Michigan Alcoholism Screening Test – Geriatric Version
The Regents of the University of Michigan/1991

	Yes
1. After drinking have you ever noticed an increase in your heart rate or beating in your chest?	
2. When talking with others, do you ever underestimate how much you actually drink?	
3. Does alcohol make you sleepy so that you often fall asleep in your chair?	
4. After a few drinks, have you sometimes not eaten or been able to skip a meal because you did not feel hungery?	
5. Does having a few drinks help decrease your shakiness or tremor?	
6. Does alcohol sometimes make it hard for you to remember parts of the day or night ?	
7. Do you have rules for yourself that you won't drink before a certain time of the day?	
8. Have you lost interest in hobbies or activities you used to enjoy?	
9. When you wake up in the morning, do you ever have trouble remembering part of the night before?	
10. Does having a drink help you sleep?	
11. Do you hide your alcohol bottles from family members?	
12. After a social gathering, have you ever felt embarrased because you drank too much?	

	Yes
13. Have you ever been concerned that drinking might be harmful to your health?	
14. Do you like to end an evening with a night cap?	
15. Did you find your drinking increased after someone close to you died?	
16. In general, would you prefer to have a few drinks at home rather than go out to social events?	
17. Are you drinking more now than in the past?	
18. Do you usually take a drink to relax or calm your nerves?	
19. Do you drink to take your mind off your problems?	
20. Have you increased your drinking after experiencing a loss in your life?	
21. Do you sometimes drive when you have had too much to drink?	
22. Has a doctor or nurse ever said they were worried or concerned about your drinking?	
23. Have you ever made rules to manage your drinking?	
24. When you feel lonely does having a drink help?	

Scoring: 5 or **more** "yes" responses indicate a problem with alcohol abuse.

Adapted from: Selzer, M.L. The Michigan Alcoholism Screening Test: the quest for a new diagnosis instrument. *Am. J. Psychiatry* 1971 **127**: 1653–1658

FALLS, GAIT AND MOBILITY DISORDERS

ASSESSING FALLS IN THE OLDER ADULT

Significance of Problem

One third of older adults living in the community report a fall or a tendency to fall. Falls, the most common cause of accidents in older adults, frequently result in fracture, especially of the hip. Hip fractures in older women have a 20-30% mortality rate at one year.

Risk factors for falls include:

- age over 80
- female gender
- history of unsteady gait
- history of mental status changes
- polypharmacy

Etiology

Falls in older adults are generally due to multifactorial causes. In most cases, reversible factors can be identified and subsequent falls prevented. Examples of causative factors include:

- Aging changes: decreased visual acuity, glare intolerance, altered depth perception, decreased auditory acuity, decreased muscle strength and/or decreased joint mobility
- Disease states: cerebrovascular disease, Parkinson's Disease, dementia, pseudodementia, cardiac dysrrhythmias, orthostatic hypotension, osteoarthritis, urinary incontinence, dehydration
- Extrinsic factors: polypharmacy, improperly fitted shoes, slippery floor surfaces, poor lighting, absence of handrails, sidewalk curbs, obstructed pathways

Diagnosis

Medical History

Because the older adult will usually not self report an isolated fall episode or even repeated falls, it is imperative to specifically question frail older adults about falling episodes. In the event of a fall history, a thorough description of the event from the patient and/or reliable source (family member caregiver) is important. This should include patient's activity at time of fall, location of fall, preceding symptoms, witness to fall and number of occurrences. Medication history should address drugs currently taken, as well as those discontinued within the last two weeks and use of over-the-counter medications. Review of systems should specifically assess for episodes of dizziness, vertigo, incontinence and cognitive changes, A comprehensive past medical history should focus on incidence of TIA's, seizure disorders, Parkinson's Disease, cataracts, glaucoma, coronary artery disease, urinary tract infections, diabetes, alcoholism and previous fractures.

Physical Exam

Particular attention should be paid to:

- blood pressure measurement in supine, sitting and standing positions to detect orthostatic hypotension
- test for visual acuity
- assessment of auditory acuity (whispered voice test),
- cardiovascular assessment to include presence of carotid bruit, cardiac rhythm and rate as well as presence of murmurs
- neurological exam to include gait, position and vibratory sense, Romberg, range of motion, muscle strength and mental status exam
- podiatric exam
- assessment for depression
- assessment for correct use of assistive devices and proper fit of shoes

Diagnostic Testing

Based on history and clinical findings, diagnostic testing may include: CBC, ESR, UA, Chem Profile, thyroid function tests, B12 and Folate, EKG, Holter monitor, CT scan of head and drug levels.

Treatment and Management

In addition to treatment of underlying medical conditions, patient's plan of care will probably include at least some of the following interventions:

- adjustment of existing medication regime as needed
- referral to physical therapy for gait training, strengthening exercises and correct use of assistive devices
- referral to podiatrist
- referral to social worker and/or occupational therapist for assessment of home environment
- patient/family teaching to address issues such as properly fitting shoes, techniques for safe position changes, toileting schedules, use of remote emergency response system
- referrals to address audiologic and/or ophthmalogical conditions.

PERFORMANCE ORIENTED MOBILITY SCREEN

Instructions: Ask the patient to perform the following maneuvers. For each maneuver, indicate the patient's performance as normal or abnormal.

ASK PATIENT TO:	NORMAL	ABNORMAL
– Sit down in chair (select chair with armrest about 16–17 inches in seat height)	★ Able to sit down in one smooth, controlled movement without using armrests	★ Sitting is not a smooth movement – falls into chair or needs armrests to guide
– Rise up from chair	★ Able to get up in one smooth movement with out using armrests	★ Uses armrests and/or moves forward in chair to propel self up; requires several attempts to get up
– Stand (about 30 seconds) after rising from chair	★ Steady, able to stand without support	★ Unsteady, loses balance
– Stand with eyes closed (about 15 seconds)	★ Steady, able to stand without support	★ Unsteady, loses balance without aid
– Stand with eyes open. Nudge on sternum with light pressure 3 times	★ Steady, needs to move feet, but able to withstand pressure and maintain balance	★ Unsteady, begins to fall
– Walk in a straight line (approximately 15 feet) at their "usual" pace, then back again	★ Gait continuous without hesitation; walks in straight line; feet clear floor ★ With Aid ★ Without Aid	★ Gait is non-continuous with deviation from straight path; feet scrape or shuffle on floor ★ With Aid ★ Without Aid
– Walk a distance of 5 feet and turn round	★ No staggering; steps are smooth, continuous ★ With Aid ★ Without Aid	★ Staggering; steps are unsteady, discontinuous ★ With Aid

Note: If the patient uses a walking aid such as a cane or walker, the walking maneuvers are tested separately (with and without aid). Indicate type of aid used:

☐ Cane   ☐ Walker   ☐ Other   ☐ None

Adapted from: Tinetti, M.E., Performance-oriented assessment of mobility problems in elderly patients. *J. Am. Geriatr. Soc.* 1996: **34**: 119-126

FALLS RISK ASSESSMENT AND PREVENTION

Step 1: Obtain history of risk factors for falls, including:

- Past history of falls
- Cognitive impairment
- Arthritis (knees, hips)
- Postural hypotension
- Gait disorder
- Incontinence
- Balance disorders (vestibular, proprioceptive, cerebellar)
- Medications (eg. psychoactive, antihypertensive, sedative drugs)

Step 2: Obtain Performance-Oriented Mobility Screen (POMS).

If POMS is NORMAL, patient is at low fall-risk. Repeat POMS if patient's condition (i.e., medical problems, medications) changes.

If POMS is ABNORMAL, patient is at fall risk. Consider one or more of the following:

Abnormality	Possible Diagnosis
Chair sitting/rising	Myopathy, arthritis, Parkinsonism, deconditioning
Standing balance	Postural hypotension, vestibular/proprioceptive dysfunction, adverse drug effect
Walking/turning	Visual, vestibular, proprioceptive, foot disorders; adverse drug effect; improper walking device or shoes
Reach up/bend down	Vestibular, vertebrobasilar, cervical dysfunction, CNS dysfunction

Step 3: Seek potentially reversible causes of fall-risk: Review medical history, including medications, for reversible causes. Perform physical examination, including comprehensive cognitive, neuro-muscular and cardiac evaluation. Obtain pertinent laboratory evaluation and diagnostic studies.

FALLS RISK ASSESSMENT AND PREVENTION

Step 4: Construct list of fall risk factors.

Step 5: Develop and implement interventions and a care plan to reduce fall risk in concert with nursing.

Write appropriate level of "activities orders" (out of bed *ad lib*; ambulation with supervision; ambulation with assistance only; complete bed rest), including use of assistive devices.

Consider frequent nursing observation (every fifteen minutes, or 24 hour observation at bed-side with private duty nursing if necessary and affordable by private pay), appropriate use of full side rails, and the appropriate use of Posey restraints as needed to prevent falls in hospital.

Reduce disorientation by appropriate environmental and reality orientation measures (such as keeping patient at nursing station during day, and lights on at night for "sundowners.".

Attempt to eliminate reversible medical causes of fall risk.

Step 6: If necessary, obtain consultation with Rehabilitation Medicine

FALLS EVALUATION AND MANAGEMENT

Step 1: Obtain fall history

["SPLATT": S–ymptoms; P–number of falls (within 3 months of admission); L–ocation; A–ctivity; T–ime (hour/date); and T–rauma.]

Obtain history of relevant complaints, medical problems, and medications. Perform physical examination, including comprehensive cognitive, neuromuscular and cardiac evaluation. Obtain pertinent laboratory evaluation and diagnostic studies.

Step 2: Do Performance-Oriented Mobility Screen (POMS).

Step 3: List differential diagnosis of fall(s).

Step 4: Obtain consultation with Physiotry for Rehabilitation if indicated

Step 5: Implement fall management plan. Consider:

> Medication review
> Neurology referral
> Physical therapy referral for gait training/exercises; walking device

Step 6: Follow-up. Obtain POMS prior to hospital discharge. If any abnormalities consider occupational therapy referral to conduct home safety evaluation.

FOOT DISORDERS

	YES	NO
1. Complaints of foot discomfort?		
2. Complaints of ambulation difficulty referable to the feet?		
3. On examination?		
Bony abnormalities		
Ulcers		
Corns/Calluses/Bunions		
Other (specify):		

If "YES" to any item, refer to Podiatry.

ASSESSMENT _____

Completed by _____

GAIT AND IMMOBILITY ASSESSMENT

The purpose of this tool is to assist in the evaluation of the patient with a mobility disorder

1. Perform a thorough history of the patient's gait problems, including
   - Test of cognitive function
   - Medication review

2. Perform a physical examination concentrating upon
   - Muscular strength and symmetry
   - Reflexes
   - Proprioception, vibratory senses
   - Foot inspection
   - Vision

3. Examine the patient's gait. Items to observe include:
   - Is the gait initiated without undue pelvic tilt?
   - Do the arms swing reciprocally and not reach out for support ?
   - Is the head held erect without spinal curvature?
   - Are the steps regular without staggering or stumbling?
   - Do the feet clear the ground with each step?
   - Does the foot strike the ground in a "heel to toe" fashion?
   - Is the step length symmetric?
   - Is the width of the stride symmetric?

4. Complete the Performance Oriented Mobility Screen

5. Consider laboratory evaluation (as indicated):
   - B12 evaluation
   - Calcium, phosphorus, alkaline phosphatase
   - TFT's
   - Drug monitoring

6. Consider the following diagnostic studies (as indicated):
   - Cervical spine films
   - Hip and knee films
   - Pelvic films
   - CT head
   - Electrophysiological studies
   - Myelography

7. ASSESSMENT

8. Consider consultation with: Rehabilitation Medicine, Geriatrician, or Neurologist as available.

Completed by _____

HEALTH MAINTENANCE

HEALTH MAINTENANCE IN THE OLDER ADULT

Significance

Health maintenance is often overlooked in the geriatric population. The perception that genetic factors are more important than environmental factors in the process of aging may play some role in this myth. However, genetic factors may only contribute about 30% of the variance in life expectancy; the other 70% appears to be related to life style factors that are preventable or manageable. Much prevention, both primary and secondary, occurs in middle age. However, with increasing longevity in our society, "preventive gerontology" is becoming increasingly important in order to promote functional life expectancy and decrease dependent life expectancy. Recent data support the notion that decreasing dependency in old age through healthy lifestyles is not only possible, but is actually occuring in the older U.S. population.

Preventive Health Guidelines for the Elderly

The need for preventive health continues unabated in old age. However, the focus of prevention shifts from preventing disease entirely to maintaining "wellness," quality of life, and the ability to function independently despite the presence of chronic illnesses.

Healthy lifestyles remain important in old age. A healthy diet can help to prevent constipation, immunoincompetence and other problems. Malnutrition is a common problem in old age that is often undetected. Up to 15% of ambulatory older patients and up to 50% of hospitalized patients are malnourished. Undernutrition is obviously an even greater problem. Malnutrition can worsen osteoporosis, impair the immune system and slow wound healing.

Exercise is of great benefit for the old, even those in their 90s and 100s. Exercise can remarkably improve an older person's daily function. Include endurance, flexibility and strength training (including weight lifting) in exercise programs. Older individuals should be seen by their primary care provider prior to beginning an exercise program.

Avoiding toxic substances such as cigarettes, alcohol and drugs (including medications) becomes even more important in old age, because the aging person has a lower tolerance. Toxic substances can have pronounced effects that might not be expressed in younger persons because older persons have less organ reserve capacity. In particular, cognitive effects of toxic substances, such as memory loss and depression, are more common in the elderly.

Preventing accidents, particularly falls, is also important in old age. The resultant injuries, such as hip fractures, can be severe. Prevention is especially effective in avoiding adverse health outcomes related to accidents in old age. For example, falls can be prevented by counselling patients about the dangers in the home of throw rugs and furniture. Driving accidents are also an important cause of morbidity and mortality in old age, and older patients should be assessed for their driving abilities (including their cognitive strengths), and counselled regarding possible ways to reduce their use of automobiles if necessary. Exercise also helps maintain balance and strength, and prevents falls and other accidents by increasing reaction time.

Osteoporosis is a common cause of loss of height and fractures in older women. Osteoporosis is preventable by hormone replacement therapy (if indicated) or other medications, a healthy diet (particularly adequate vitamin D and calcium), and exercise.

Maintaining mental health is vital to quality of life and independence in old age. Senility or dementia is not a normal part of aging, and may be treatable. Depression is also a common treatable problem in old age. Socialization, vigorous mental activity, physical exercise, a healthy diet, avoidance of toxic substances including medications, all contribute to robust mental health.

Cancer screening remains important in the elderly, although some aspects of screening change from the middle age adult population because of a change in the epidemiology of some cancers. Mammography, colorectal screening, and prostate cancer screening remain important, as are preventive strategies such as avoiding smoking.

Vaccinations remain effective in the elderly and should be given on a regular basis. The primary vaccines employed include influenza (yearly), pneumovax, and tetanus (every ten years). In particular, most elderly individuals are not immunized to tetanus, and as a result the prevalence rate of tetanus is highest among the old.

With proper preventive measures, a productive and successful old age is an achieveable goal for most older persons.

PREVENTIVE CARE GUIDELINES FOR OLDER ADULTS

This tool provides the tests that are generally recommended for annual preventive health care in the elderly. These guidelines were prepared, in part, based on the recommendations of the United States Preventive Services Task Force.

	Age 65-74	Age 75 +
Physical examination:		
Blood pressure	annually	
Weight	annually	
Mouth and teeth	annually	
Breasts	annually	
Digital rectal exam	annually	
Vision	if indicated	annually
Tests:		
Mammography	every 1–2 years	no recommendation
PAP smear	every 2 years; if two recent exams normal, then discontinue	as indicated
Stool for blood	annually	annually
Vaccinations:		
Tetanus	every ten years	
Pneumococcal pneumonia	once	
Influenza	annually	
Counselling:		
Nutrition	annually	
Exercise	annually	
Medication Review	annually	
Advanced Directives	review annually	
Osteoporosis	every five years	
Hearing	if necessary	annually
Ability to function independently in the community	if necessary	annually
Mental Health (memory and mood)	if necessary	annually
Injury Prevention (falls and driving)	if necessary	annually
Smoking and Alcohol	if necessary	

HEALTH MAINTENANCE

This tool provides a listing of health maintenance items that may be assessed during ambulatory care. The tool also facilitates the transfer of health maintenance information to the medical record for followup. Recommendations on the frequency of these examinations is not given; many of the items may be considered optional by the clinician.

	DATE OF EXAM	RESULTS	COMMENTS
1.EXAMINATIONS			
A. Vision			
B. Dental			
C. Audiology			
D. Podiatry			
F. Cognitive			
G. Other			
II. LABORATORIES			
A. B12/Folate			
B. TFT's			
C. VDRL			
D. ECG			
E. PPD			
F. Stool for occult blood			
G. Other			
III. PROCEDURES			
A. Mammogram			
B. Sigmoidoscopy			
C. PAP Smear			
D. Other			
IV. IMMUNIZATIONS			
A. Pneumovax			
B. Influenza			
C. Tetanus/Diphtheria			
D. Other			
V. COUNSELLING			
A. Tobacco Use			
B. Alcohol Use			
C. Medication Use			
D. Sexual Activities			
E. Dietary Habits			
F. Exercise			
G. Driving/Seatbelt Use			
H. Falls			
K. Osteoporosis			
L. Other			

Completed by _____   Date _____

IMMUNOCOMPETENCE
ASSESSMENT

IMMUNOCOMPETENCE ASSESSMENT

Introduction

Immunodeficiency is one of the major geriatric syndromes which are generally multifactorial in etiology. Immune function declines with age and has been extensively investigated. The primary changes in immune function occur in the cellular immune system. In particular, T-cell function declines with age. These changes in T cell function are responsible, at least in part, for the increased susceptibility to infection and complications from infections, such as bacteremia, sepsis and mortality, which occurs in old age. The altered T cell function may affect humoral immunity as well, although primary alterations in B cell function may also occur. One result of altered cellular immunity is decreased capacity to fight or contain intracellular viral and bacterial infections, and reactivation infections, such as herpes zoster and tuberculosis, may result. Whether the decline in immune function with old age results in an increased susceptibility to cancer and autoimmune diseases remains unclear. Some evidence suggests that a decline in immune surveillance and other changes in immune function may contribute to the increased susceptibility to cancer that occurs in old age. Finally, while autoimmune phenomena, such as low affinity autoantibodies to DNA and rheumatoid factor, increase with age, their relationship to autoimmune disease is also unclear. However, pernicious anemia and autoimmune thyroid disease are clearly age-related autoimmune diseases associated with increased titers of circulating autoantibodies.

As with other geriatric syndromes, the primary task of the clinician is to distinguish between the effects of normal aging and possible secondary causes which may be reversible. The most common cause of secondary acquired immune deficiency in the elderly is malnutrition. Malnutrition mimics, in most aspects, and exacerbates the effects of aging on immune competence. For example, malnutrition leads to immune deficiency, increasing suseptibility to infection, which is the most common cause of death due to malnutrition. In many instances, it is likely that the old man's friend, pneumonia, may be preventable if nutritional status could be normalized.

Other causes of secondary immune dysfunction include medications which may alter immune function, such as steroids, nonsteroidal antiinflammatory medications, and a host of other medications. HIV infection also may occur in the elderly and should be considered.

Evaluation of the patient for immune competence

Immune competence can be evaluated rather simply by the clinician. Evaluation of cellular immunity is easily done by employing laboratory tests and skin testing. Circulating levels of lymphocytes, including most classes (T and B cells) and subclasses, polymorphonuclear leucocytes, and monocytes, do not change with age. In particular, low levels of circulating lymphocytes are abnormal and an indication of immune dysfunction. Delayed type hypersensitivity is a reliable indicator of cellular immune function. Impaired delayed type hypersenitivity, or anergy, correlates robustly with outcomes such as mortality in the elderly. Evaluation of the humoral immune system is equally simple. Total immunoglobulin levels generally do not change with age. IgG levels may actually increase. Markedly increased levels of immunoglobulins, either monoclonal or polyclonal, are a sign of immune dysfunction in aging as well, suggesting multiple myeloma, chronic infections, and other illnesses.

Management and Treatment of Immune Deficiency in Old Age

Once a diagnosis of acquired immune deficiency has been established, an evaluation for reversible causes should be pursued. The evaluation of malnutrition is described elsewhere in this volume. Protein-calorie malnutrition, but also specific vitamin (such as vitamin B12, vitamin E and others) and mineral (such as zinc) deficiencies, may cause impaired immune function. Replacement therapy may reverse immune deficiency in these cases and prevent subsequent morbidity and even mortality. A complete medication review should also be performed to discover medications which may impair immune function. In patients with severe lymphopenia, appropriate risk factors may be sought for HIV infection and a T4/T8 ratio performed. It should be noted that a number of acute and chronic diseases may impair immune function and elderly persons with multiple comorbidities may suffer anergy as a result. For these individuals, control of the underlying comorbidities is most important to retain immune function.

Strategies to enhance immune function remain an active area of research. Hormones, vitamins and a variety of other medications have been advocated as immune enhancers to reverse aging of the immune system or to enhance immune function in patients with chronic diseases. To date, none of these strategies has been proven effective. Maintenance of a healthy diet and lifestyle, including exercise, are probably the simplest and most effective methods for maintaining immune function in late life.

Finally, older individuals generally respond adequately to vaccination. Routine vaccination remains an effective strategy for preventing infection, particularly pneumonia and tetanus, in the elderly. Although frail, anergic individuals may fail to respond to vaccinations, no recommendations can be made at this time for advocating enhanced dosaging or frequency of vaccinations in this population.

IMMUNOCOMPETENCE ASSESSMENT

The purpose of this tool is to assist in the evaluation of the patient's state of immune competence

I. Evaluation of the cellular immune system:

     A. Total white cell count _____

     B. Total lymphocyte count _____
         (mild to moderate lymphopenia = <1200 cells/mm^3

         severe lymphopenia = < 900 cells/mm^3)

If severe lymphopenia is present, consider T_4/T_8 ratio. If this ratio is depressed, and appropriate risk factors are present (e.g. history of transfusion, drug abuse, or homosexuality) consider an HIV test

     C. Delayed type skin hypersensitivity testing

PPD Status:	Date
a) Positive	
b) Negative	
c) Non-reactive	
d) Unknown _____	

If PPD status is negative or unknown, administer the PPD(5TU). This test can be done if: a) the patient has no history of active tuberculosis and b) the patient is currently not on any anti-tuberculin medication.

If, at 48-72 hours, the area of induration is > or = 4mm consider the test to be positive and evaluate further as indicated. If, at 48-72 hours, the area of induration is < 4mm but there is some area of induration, repeat the test at 7-21 days. If, at 48-72 hours, there is no area of induration, consider the test to be non-reactive and proceed to D.

IMMUNOCOMPETENCE ASSESSMENT

    D.   To further assess delayed type skin hypersensitivity:

    1.   Repeat the PPD at least 7 days after the initial test

    2.   Administer the following skin tests:

	Date	Result (mm)
Candida		
Mumps		
Coccidioidin		
Histoplasmin		
Tetanus		
Other		

An area of induration of > or = 4mm for any of these tests constitutes a positive response. If all tests are negative, consider the patient anergic for delayed type skin hypersensitivity.

II. Evaluation of the <u>humoral immune system</u>

    A. Total globulins (may use total protein – albumin)
    B. Serum protein electrophoresis (if globulins are elevated, to evaluate for myeloma)
    C. Specific antibody titers may be measured (eg. anti-tetanus toxoid, isoagglutinins, etc.)

III. Immunization Status up to date?

    a) Influenza   Yes/No
    b) Pneumovax   Yes/No
    c) Tetanus(within 10 years)   Yes/No
    d) Diphtheria   Yes/No
    e) Other

<u>Assessment:</u> :

    Normal _____

    If anergic and/or lymphopenic, consider acquired immunodeficiency secondary to :

    malnutrition _____
    medications _____
    other (HIV, acute or chronic illness) _____
    If indicated, refer for Clinical Immunology consultation.

Completed by _____

INCONTINENCE ASSESSMENT

ASSESSMENT OF FECAL INCONTINENCE IN THE OLDER ADULT

Significance of Problem

As many as 25% of hospitalized older adults and up to 50% of those in nursing homes experience fecal incontinence, the inability to control defecation. Fecal incontinence leads to social isolation and dependency for the older adult while placing the individual at greater risk for institutionalization.

Etiology

The major causes of fecal incontinence in the older adult are:

- fecal impaction
- laxative misuse or abuse
- neurological disorders such as dementia and cerebrovascular disease
- colon-rectal diseases such as irritable bowel syndrome, rectal prolapse, diabetic neuropathy, carcinoma, anal fissures or fistulas

Diagnosis

Medical History

It is essential to have an understanding of the patient's normal bowel patterns when assessing the problem of fecal incontinence. Specific questions regarding fecal incontinence include chronicity and frequency of problem, precipitating factors and associated symptoms such as abdominal cramping, urgency, presence of blood or mucus in stool.

Obtain a detailed medication history with attention to use of over-the-counter laxatives and use of enemas. A dietary history including daily fluid intake pattern is also valuable.

Past medical history should include all surgical procedures as well as number of pregnancies with type of delivery.

Physical Exam

Abdominal and rectal exam are essential. In addition, assessment of mental status will help to establish etiology of fecal incontinence and appropriate course of treatment.

Treatment and Management

Treatment options are based on etiology of fecal incontinence, the patient's level of understanding and availability of caregiver support.

If impaction is cause of fecal incontinence, interventions to prevent further episodes of constipation should be implemented after removal of fecal impaction. Increased fluid and fiber intake are helpful, as well as an increase in level of activity. Lactulose (30–45 ml/daily) can be utilized on a long term basis to lessen further episodes of constipation.

When dementia or a similar neurological disorder is cause of fecal incontinence, interventions to prevent constipation are essential in conjunction with the establishment of toileting schedules to meet the patient's pattern of defecation.

Educating the older adult about age related changes of the gastoinstestional tract and the correct use of laxatives and enemas is critical when the problem of fecal incontinence is due to laxative misuse. Positive reinforcement is important as the patient strives to break old habits and implement correct health practices.

Biofeedback is a treatment modality producing positive results when the patient has no cognitive impairment, is motivated and has rectal sensation.

Surgical intervention may be indicated for correction of severe rectal prolapse and carcinoma causing fecal incontinence.

When fecal incontinence is due to neuropathy, a regime with a consistent toileting schedule for defecation and a low fiber intake will help to lessen fecal incontinence.

While the problem of fecal incontinence is being addressed, attention should be paid to personal hygiene to prevent skin breakdown and urinary tract infections.

ASSESSMENT OF FECAL INCONTINENCE

The purpose of this tool is to assist in the evaluation of the patient with fecal incontinence.

A. From gathered history, from physical examination, and from noninvasive testing (KUB, etc.) does there appear to be a structural abnormality of the colon?

        If "YES", then refer for appropriate therapy.

        If "NO", then proceed to B.

B. Is there a fecal impaction?

        If "YES", then:
- Disimpact
- Evaluate for need for hydration
- Evaluate for need for enemas
- Consider a high fiber diet
- Consider bulkforming agents
- Evaluate patient's exercise capabilities
- Consider toilet training
- Evaluate medications for possible causative agents

        If "NO", then:
Maximize medical treatment
- exploit the gastrocolic reflex
- use bulkforming agents
- consider the use of Keigle exercises
- consider the use of enemas
- consider the use of anti-diarrheal agents

C. If there is a poor response to the above measures, consider a GI consultant for further evaluation.

D. If no organic cause is found, consider FUNCTIONAL INCONTINENCE if moderate to severe cognitive impairment is present.

ASSESSMENT OF CAUSE OF FECAL INCONTINENCE _____

Completed by _____

ASSESSMENT OF URINARY INCONTINENCE

Significance of Problem

Urinary incontinence, the involuntary loss of urine, is experienced by up to 30% community dwelling older adults and 50% of those residing in nursing homes. Urinary incontinence can result in loss of self esteem and independence, social isolation and depression.

Physiologically, the older adult with urinary incontinence is prone to urinary tract infections with urosepsis, falls with subsequent fractures and skin breakdown with decubitus ulcer development. Frequently, urinary incontinence is the major cause for long term institutionalization. It is estimated that over $15 billion is spent annually in managing incontinence.

Etiology

Risk factors for urinary incontinence include:

- advanced age
- female gender
- parity
- infection such as urinary tract and atrophic vaginitis
- medications, including: diuretics, anticholinergics, psychotropics and narcotics
- hormonal changes
- hyperglycemia
- alcohol abuse
- fecal impaction
- disease states such as dementia, cerebrovascular accident , delirium, diabetes, congestive heart failure.

Diagnosis

Medical History

Because many older adults assume that loss of urinary control is a normal process of aging, they often do not initiate discussion about incontinence during the medical history. Since urinary incontinence affects up to 20% of women over the age of 80 and 5% of women over the age of 65, the health care provider should routinely ask direct questions about the presence of urinary incontinence for all women over the age of 75. Questions about incontinence should also be asked of men at risk (such as those with prostate disease), and men and women in whom there is a high index of suspicion (such as individuals who present with the odor of urine on their clothing).

If the patient does experience involuntary loss of urine, a detailed history should include: duration, frequency, precipitating factors, amount of urine lost, associated symptoms such as burning, nocturia and hesitancy, pattern of fluid intake and alterations in bowel pattern or sexual function. The clinician should review all medications including over-the-counter drugs for possibly contributing to incontinence. Past medical history should include surgical procedures that may affect the urinary tract and number of pregnancies.

Physical Exam

Essential elements of the physical exam in the older adult with urinary incontinence include palpation and percussion of the abdomen, rectal, pelvic exam in women, and prostate exam in men. A comprehensive neurological exam includes gait assessment as well as mental status exam. A functional assessment should assess the impact of incontinence on daily function.

Diagnostic Testing

Urinalysis, urine culture and blood chemistries to include BUN, creatinine, electrolytes and glucose should be done. Post voiding residual by catheterization is a simple procedure that is very helpful in the differential diagnosis of incontinence. Ultrasound may also be of value to complete initial diagnostic process.

Treatment and Management

Treatment options will be based on the type of urinary incontinence, the patient's level of comprehension, degree of motivation and accessibility of caregiver support.

Refer to the following table for classifications of urinary incontinence, presenting clinical signs and examples of treatment options.

Indwelling urethral catheters for urinary incontinence are indicated: 1) on a short term basis in the care of patients with severe decubitus ulcers whose healing may be affected by constant soiling and moisture, or 2) in patients with obstructive disease. Condom catheters are sometimes helpful for male patients, but skin breakdown may occur as a result of their use. Pads and special undergarments may be selected based on the patient's individual needs.

It is critical that health care professionals recognize that incontinence is not a normal process of aging and teach older adults that it is a condition that is often reversible and warrants a thorough assessment. In most cases urinary incontinence can be cured or at least improved.

Classification	Etiology	Clinical Signs	Treatment Options
stress incontinence	outlet incompetence	leakage of small to moderate amount of urine as intrabdominal pressure increases, occurs with coughing, sneezing, bending, lifting, laughing	Pelvic floor exercises for men and women★; toileting schedules; hormone replacement therapy; surgical correction
urge incontinence	detrusor instability or hyperflexia, common in urinary tract infection, neurological disorders such as cerebrovascular accident	uninhibited bladder contractions cause loss of moderate amount of urine, occurs at several hour intervals	treat urinary tract infection; implement bladder training★★ Anticholinergics, such as oxybutnin and propantheline, reduce involuntary bladder contraction. Watch for dry mouth, constipation, confusion, blurred vision
overflow incontinence	outlet obstruction or underactive detrusor seen with spinal cord lesion, medications, prostatic hypertrophy, fecal impaction	overdistended bladder cannot empty, leads to nearly constant loss of urine	treat underlying conditions: constipation, prostatic hypertrophy; intermittent catheterization
functional incontinence	environmental factors or underlying medical conditions such as dementia, osteoarthritis	loss of large amounts of urine	address underlying environmental issues e.g. easier access to toilet facilities with improved lighting, raised toilet seats, grab bars, easily removable clothing; restrict bedtime fluids; assistive devices to increase ambulation skills

★ patient should be taught to sustain muscle contraction for up to 10 seconds in sets of 10 contractions. Sets should be repeated three to five times a day. Most favorable results are achieved by women 75 years of age or younger. Patients should be encouraged to continue exercises even after incontinence has stopped.

★★ scheduled urination every 30-60 minutes initially for one week, increase by 30 minute intervals each week thereafter as number of incontinent episodes decrease with ultimate goal of 2-3 hour intervals.

ASSESSMENT OF URINARY INCONTINENCE

The purpose of this tool is to assist in the evaluation and treatment of urinary incontinence.

Initial investigation:

- History including type, pattern, associated symptoms and duration of incontinence, and medication review
- Physical (including bladder, pelvic, rectal, prostate and neurologic);
- Laboratory (including urinalysis and culture)
- Special tests:

    1) 24 hour voiding record to assess voiding pattern (urge, stress, overflow, reflex and functional)

    2) Have the patient cough with a full bladder (preferably while standing):

    a) if there is loss of urine, consider detrusor instability and/or urethral sphincter incompetence. Pursue further with bedside manometrics, if indicated.

    b) if there is no loss of urine, check a postvoid residual volume. If PVR is >150 ml and no fecal impaction or other mass lesion is present, then consider obstruction, neurogenic bladder or other causes. If PVR is < 150 ml, then consider detrusor instability and other causes.

For transient incontinence: Consider causes [**DIAPPERS**]:

D – Delirium
I – Infection
A – Atrophic vaginitis/urethritis
P – Pharmaceuticals (particularly sedative/hypnotics, anticholinergics, "loop" diurectics, alpha agonists and antagonists, and calcium channel blockers)
P – Psychological, particularly depression
E – Endocrine (hyperglycemia, hypercalcemia)
R – Restricted mobility
S – Stool impaction

ASSESSMENT OF URINARY INCONTINENCE

<u>For established incontinence</u>: Consider categories of cases:

- Detrusor overactivity
- Detrusor underactivity
- Outlet incompetence
- Outlet obstruction

Urodynamics and Consultation

If diagnosis is not determined after initial investigation, consider consultation and urodynamics evaluation (possibly including cystometry, urethral profilometry, uroflowmetry, electromyography, and appropriate radiographics and ultrasonographic examination).

Consider consultation with genitourinary service when indicated.

ASSESSMENT OF CAUSE OF URINARY INCONTINENCE

Completed by: _____

NUTRITIONAL ASSESSMENT

NUTRITIONAL ASSESSMENT OF THE OLDER ADULT

Significance of Problem

Malnutrition in older adults is a serious and sometimes fatal disorder that is often not diagnosed. For example, although malnutrition may effect up to 40% of hospitalized elderly patients, it is undiagnosed in more than half of all cases. Types of malnutrition include protein-calorie malnutrition, marasmus and specific vitamin and mineral deficiencies, all of which can cause morbidity and mortality. Malnutrition is a predisposing factor to infection, e.g. pneumonia, skin breakdown or poor wound healing, altered mental status, increased incidence of falls with subsequent fracture and altered drug metabolism in the older adult. Therefore, it is a condition that warrants a thorough medical assessment.

Etiology

Many factors put an older adult at risk for poor nutritional health and/or malnutrition. Included are those related to:

- *Medical Conditions:* dementia, depression, Parkinson's Disease, Osteoarthritis, CVA, malabsorption syndromes, alcohol misuse, cancer, congestive heart failure.
- *Psychosocial Issues:* living alone, limited access to food (limited finances, lack of transportation, limited cooking facilities), cultural preferences
- *Physiological Factors:* decreased vision, decreased sense of smell and/or taste, poor dentition, polypharmacy (producing anorexia)
- *Educational Issues:* limited understanding of nutritional needs, with inadequate consumption of fruits, vegetables, milk products and grains.

Diagnosis

Medical History

To assess for malnutrition, it is important to determine recent unintentional weight loss, for example, 5% or more of body weight in one month; 10% or more of body weight in 6 months. Inquire about recent illnesses and/or hospitalizations, as well as comorbidity, such as, thyroid disease and cancer.

Obtain a minimum of a 24 hour diet recall from the patient and/or reliable source(family member care giver). Not only should this include the types and quantities of foods consumed but also the settings in which foods are consumed. Fluid intake should also be assessed. In addition, it is important to note not only current prescription medication use, but also use of over-the-counter medications. It is not uncommon for an older adult to utilize vitamins, minerals and laxatives in inappropriate amounts, altering absorption of nutrients. Inquire about changes in appetite, dental problems, use of alcohol, altered mental status and/ or feelings of sadness. To complete this process, obtain information about the individual's functional capabilities, as well as socio-economic factors, as they relate to food acquisition and meal preparation.

Physical Exam

Obtain body mass index (BMI: weight[kg.]/height[cm]2). When this is not appropriate because of the patient's immobility, obtain knee/height measurement. Perform anthropometric measurements when available. Attention should be given to color and condition of skin as well as the degree of muscle tone. Exam of the mouth for presence of stomatitis and condition of teeth is important. Neurological exam should include testing to assess cognitive function and to check for presence of depression.

Diagnostic Testing

Laboratory studies to facilitate in diagnosis of malnutrition include:
    Serum albumin
    Serum cholesterol
    Total lymphocyte count

A diagnosis of malnutrition is generally made by the presence of two of the following criteria:

1.   Ideal Body Weight <90% or Body Mass Index <22
2.   Serum Albumin <3.5. Serum cholesterol <2.5 g/dl indicates severe malnutrition and is associated with markedly increased morbidity and mortality in the hospitalized patient
3.   Total lymphocyte count <1500 cells/mm^3 (or otherwise corrected for local laboratory values)

Treatment and Management

Based on history, physical findings and diagnostic screen, several treatment options are appropriate for the older adult who suffers malnutrition or is at risk for malnutrition. Pharmacological interventions are available to address conditions such as vitamin deficiencies, depression and hypothyroidism contributing to the state of malnutrition,

Referral to other members of the health care team will be essential to address functional issues contributing to the problem of malnutrition. A social worker referral will assist the patient with procuring community resources such as Meals-on-Wheels, Adult Day Care, food stamps, community nutrition sites, home health aide services, transportation services, or seeking an alternative living environment. These interventions will help to remove socio-economic barriers to good nutrition.

Recommendation for follow-up with a nutritionist will help to address knowledge deficits the older adult may have about meal planning. Occupational therapy referral is appropriate if the patient's poor nutrition is related to lack of manual dexterity and/or need for assistive devices for preparation or ingestion of food.

Referral to nursing staff will help caregiver to manage problems related to inadequate intake of food in the cognitively impaired patient.

Malnutrition due to poor dentition or ill-fitting dentures warrants a dental referral.

In addition, the use of oral nutritional supplementation should be considered for an individual with BMI<22, Serum albumin <3.5, or inadequate dietary intake.

Enteral feeding via nasogastric or PEG may be appropriate for end stage patients with dementing illnesses, especially if the desire for aggressive therapies is documented in an advance directive.

Total parental nutrition should be considered for individuals being prepared for surgical procedures.

NUTRITIONAL ASSESSMENT

Risk for Poor Nutrition: The Nutrition Screening Initiative

This tool assist in the identification of individuals who are at risk for poor nutrition, which may be precusor of malnutrition.

	Yes
I have an illness or condition that made me change the kind and/or amount of food I eat	2
I eat fewer than 2 meals per day	3
I eat few fruits or vegetables, or milk products	2
I have 3 or more drinks of beer, liquor or wine almost every day	2
I have tooth or mouth problems that make it hard for me to eat	2
I don't always have enough money to buy the food I need	4
I eat alone most of the time	1
I take 3 or more different prescribed or over-the-counter drugs a day	1
Without wanting to, I have lost or gained 10 pounds in the last 6 months	2
I am not always physically able to shop, cook and/or feed myself	2
Total	

Scoring:

0-2: Normal

3-5: Moderate risk for poor nutrition. Improved eating habits and lifestyle are indicated. Patients should be referred to local senior programs that assist in providing nutrition to seniors.

6 or more: high nutritional risk. The patient should be seen by a physician, dietician or social worker to intervene to improve nutritional health.

NUTRITIONAL ASSESSMENT

Risk for Poor Nutrition: The Nutrition Screening Initiative

The Nutrition Checklist: *DETERMINE*	PRESENT
Disease (consider chronic conditions which affect eating)	
Eating poorly (evaluate overall diet for nutritional content)	
Tooth loss/mouth pain	
Economic hardship	
Reduced social contact	
Multiple medicines (consider drug effects on appetite including taste, constipation, diarrhea, nausea, confusion)	
Involuntary weight loss/gain	
Needs asssistance in self care	
Elder years above age 80 (increases risk)	

Adapted from The Nutrition Screening Initiative: The original tool was developed by The Nutrition Screening Initiative (American Academy of Family Physicians, the American Dietetic Association and the National Council on Aging), and was funded through a grant from Ross Laboratories.

NUTRITIONAL ASSESSMENT

The purpose of this tool is to assess the nutritional status of the patient and to identify those patients who have existing evidence of malnutrition or are at risk for the development of malnutrition.

Please check the following

1. Historical Information	
A. Greatest height (at age 20)	
B. History of weight loss (>10 lbs. in last 6 months)	
C. Complaints of change in appetite	
2. Average 24 hour calorie count	
Is this sufficient to maintain or increase the patient's weight?	
3. Nutritional Parameters	
A. Weight	
Is this <90% ideal body weight for age?	
B. Serum albumin (abnormal if < 3.5 mg/dl)	
C. Hemoglobin	
D. TIBC	
E. Transferrin [estimate by (0.8 X TIBC) – 43]	
F. Total lymphocyte count	
G. Cholesterol	
H. Other	
4. Immunocompetence Status (refer to separate protocol)	
Normal or abnormal	
5. Anthropometric Parameters	
A. Body Mass Index (weight/height^2) (<22 is abnormal)	
B. Triceps skinfold	
C. Midarm circumference	

ASSESSMENT

Consider consultation with nutritionist

Completed by _____

ORAL and DENTAL ASSESSMENT

1. Complaints of oral problems? Describe

2. **Dental Screening Initiative Instrument:**

	If yes, point value
Dry mouth	2
Eating difficulty	1
No recent dental care (within 2 years)	1
Tooth or mouth pain	2
Alteration or change in food selection	1
Lesions, sores or lumps in the mouth	2

If the patient scores more than 2 points, referral for dental care is recommended.

3. Problems with dentures or bridgework? _____

4. On examination:

A. Abnormal hygiene:
B. Abnormal lips:
C. Abnormal mucosa:
D. Abnormal teeth:
E. Abnormal gums:
F. Abnormal tongue:
G. Abnormal Palate:
H. Other:

If "YES" to any item, refer for dental care, Oral Surgery or otolaryngology as appropriate for further consultation.

FEEDING DISORDER ASSESSMENT

The purpose of this worksheet is to assist in the evaluation and treatment of the patient with a feeding disorder.

A. Historical

        Y N   1. Has the patient had a loss of 10% of their ideal body weight over the last 6 months?

        Y N   2. Does the patient complain of a poor appetite or does the caregiver complain of poor eating habits?

        Y N   3. Does the caregiver complain that the patient often chokes, gags, or potentially aspirates food while eating?

B. Medication Review (particularly those medications which may cause dyspepsia or dysgeusia (disorders of taste))

    1. _____   4. _____

    2. _____   5. _____

    3. _____   6. _____

C. Medical conditions which may interfere with a patient's feeding abilities, which may contribute to weight loss, or may cause a feeding disorder

    1. _____   4. _____

    2. _____   5. _____

    3. _____   6. _____

	Comment
D. **Physical Examination**	
1. Oral cavity	
2. Gag reflex	
3. Upper extremity function	
4. Observed feeding behavior	
E. **Other**	
1. ADL score	
2. Body Mass Index	
3. Serum albumin	
4. Lymphocyte count	
5. 24 hour caloric intake	
6. **Other**	

ASSESSMENT

If evidence is found of a feeding disorder consider consultation with the following as appropriate: Medical Nutrition Team, Speech Therapy, Occupational Therapy, or Gastroenterology.

Completed by _____

OSTEOPOROSIS AND METABOLIC BONE DISEASE

OSTEOPOROSIS and METABOLIC BONE DISEASE

Significance

Osteoporosis is a debilitating disease that affects about 25% of women, results in approximately 1.3 million fractures yearly in the United States, generating as much as $10 billion in health care costs for the treatment of these fractures. While these costs are primarily for hip fractures, wrist, vertebral and other fractures can be equally debilitating and affect quality of life. Hip fractures may be fatal in up to 20% of women over the age of 75, due to loss of ambulation, immobility, and functional decline. Vertebral fractures, resulting in loss of height, may cause chronic, sometimes severe back pain. In the end stage severe case, loss of spinal height may cause ribs to literally rub on the pelvis, presenting as chronic, sometimes severe, abdominal pain and impaired function.

Assessment

Postmenopausal osteoporosis, and the resultant fractures, is generally a preventable disorder with appropriate assessment and therapy. Therefore, recognition of the problem by physicians, assessment and diagnosis are crucial to preventing the comorbidities of osteoporosis.

All postmenopausal women should have at least one evaluation and counselling session regarding osteoporosis. The session should include a review of existing risk factors, counselling on positive and negative lifestyle factors, and consideration of estrogen replacement therapy or other therapies.

Risk factors include those which affect peak bone mass attainment, and those which cause bone loss. These factors include race (caucasian and oriental women being at greater risk), early estrogen deficiency, calcium and/or vitamin D deficiency, lifestyle risk factors including lack of exercise or immobilization, smoking, excessive use of alcohol or caffeine; and medications or prior or concurrent diseases.

Bone mineral density is preferably assessed by dual energy X-ray absorptiometry. Densitometry is generally indicated for women who are considering long term estrogen replacement therapy for whom the results of densitometry would influence their decision. For example, some women may only wish to take estrogen replacement therapy if bone densitometry reveals low bone density.

During the evaluation, consideration should be given to metabolic bone disease and secondary causes of osteoporosis in women with severe osteoporosis and associated laboratory or other abnormalities. These include various endocrinopathies such as hyperparathyroidism, hypercortisolism, and hyperthyroidism, as well as drugs (particularly steriods, excess thyroid replacement or inappropriate thyroxine usage, heparin, phenytoin, excess aluminum containing antacids), and various chronic conditions such as renal failure, malabsorption syndromes, osteomalacia, and prolonged immobility.

Treatment and Management

Hormone replacement therapy with estrogen and, when indicated progesterone, is generally the treatment of choice for postmenopausal osteoporosis. For each woman, the benefits of estrogen replacement therapy must be weighed against the risks, primarily endometrial cancer and probably some increase in the risk of breast cancer, as well as the inconvenience of menstrual bleeding, although the latter may be amerliorated by newer, continuous estrogen/progesterone combination therapy. The most common problem with estrogen replacement therapy in the prevention of osteoporosis is long term compliance. Less than 25% of women who might benefit from estrogen replacement therapy are currently taking it and this percentage declines significantly with the number of years from menopause.

For women who are unable or unwilling to take estrogen replacement therapy, calcitonin and biphosphonates such as alendronate are reasonable alternatives, particularly in women with established disease as demonstrated by dual photon densitometry.

Strategies for the prevention of osteoporosis include appropriate exercise and diet, with adequate calcium and vitamin D intake, and avoidance of risk factors such as excess alcohol, drugs that may cause or exacerbate osteoporosis, and other factors. Counselling of the patient on a periodic basis is crucial to maintaining compliance with healthy lifestyles that can reduce the rate of bone loss through dietary deficiency states or by drugs and other factors. However, these factors alone will not slow the rate of bone loss in the postmenopausal women who is not treated with estrogen or other medications. It should be noted that, even in elderly woman who are years beyond menopause, estrogen replacement therapy may result in some restoration of bone density and reduction of fracture susceptibility.

Management of vertebral fractures is generally conservative and involves primarily bed rest and analgesis, followed by physical therapy as indicated. Other fractures generally require orthopedic intervention, followed by physical therapy as indicated to restore prior functional abilities.

OSTEOPOROSIS AND METABOLIC BONE DISEASE ASSESSMENT

This checklist is designed to assist in the recognition and evaluation of the geriatric patient who may be at risk for the complications associated with osteoporosis and other metabolic bone diseases.

RISK FACTORS

Women of British, Northern European, Scandinavian, Chinese, or Japanese descent
Poor calcium intake either because of malabsorption or lactose intolerance
Protein calorie malnutrition
A relatively high dietary intake of protein
Thin body habitus
Relative immobility and lack of weightbearing exercise
A history of alcoholism
A history of smoking
A history of heavy caffeine use
A history of gastrectomy
Onset of menopause before the age of 45 or an early surgical menopause
Use of medications that induce the calcium loss including:
Glucocorticoids, Anticonvulsants, Thyroid preparations, INH, Tetracycline, Lasix, Heparin

HISTORY

A history of fractures of: vertebral bodies, femoral head, radius, or other site
A history of back pain
A history of loss of height

PHYSICAL EXAMINATION

Height _____ Tallest past height _____ Presence of "Dowager's hump" Yes No

LABORATORY TESTS TO CONSIDER

Serum calcium	SPEP
Phosphorus	UPEP
Alkaline phosphatase	TFT's
BUN/ Creatinine	PTH
Glucose	Urine cAMP
LFT's	25-OH-Vitamin D

OSTEOPOROSIS AND METABOLIC BONE DISEASE ASSESSMENT (continued)

LABORATORY TESTS TO CONSIDER

24 hr. urine calcium

Fasting spot urine calcium

Bone biopsy

Testosterone

Bone scan

RADIOLOGIC TESTS

Plain films of:
- Spine
- Wrists

Bone densitometry (indicated if):
- The decision for instituting long-term therapy will be affected by the densitometry results
- Screening for persons with major risk factors of:
  - prolonged amenorrhea
  - early menopause
  - gastric or small bowel resection
  - chronic treatment with glucocorticoids, anticonvulsants, or thyroid preparations

ASSESSMENT

Primary or senile osteoporosis

Secondary osteoporosis (circle as appropriate)
- Hyperadrenocortism
- Hyperthyroidism
- Hypogonadism
- Immobility
- Diabetes mellitus
- Alcoholism
- Chronic anticonvulsant use
- Chronic aluminum containing antacid use
- Chronic heparin use
- Chronic renal failure
- Metastatic bone disease
- Liver disease
- Methotrexate therapy
- Scurvy
- Malabsorption Syndrome
- COPD
- Rheumatoid arthritis
- Systemic mastocytosis
- Osteogenesis imperfecta
- Hyperparathyroidism
- Osteomalacia
- Multiple Myeloma

If indicated, consider consultation with the Osteoporsis and Metabolic Bone Disease Clinic, endocrinology or other specialist.

Completed by _____

POLYPHARMACY

POLYPHARMACY IN THE OLDER ADULT

Significance of Problem

Polypharmacy, the use of multiple prescription and over-the-counter medications, results in drug interactions, adverse drug reactions, and patient non-compliance. Up to 15% of hospitalizations of elderly are the consequence of adverse drug reactions and as many as 45% of hospital readmissions are related to problems of medication use.

Etiology

Contributing factors to polypharmacy in older adults span many issues. Older adults experience multiple diagnoses with atypical presentation and increased severity of illness frequently resulting in use of multiple medications. A limited knowledge of correct medication administration by the older adult results in noncompliance, use of discontinued medications, under-reporting of medication use to each health care provider, over use of over-the counter drugs and utilization of services of multiple health care providers and pharmacies. Finally, failure to incorporate principles of geriatric pharmacology into practice by the health care provider contributes to polypharmacy.

Diagnosis

Medical History

A complete drug history including not only prescription drugs but also over-the-counter medications is imperative. Ideally, this is completed by a brown bag drug review. This allows the health care provider not only to visualize each medication in its original container, but also to assess the older adults implementation of the drug regimen.

Physical Exam

Several components of the physical exam will lend meaningful information to the older adult's ongoing abilities to implement drug regimen correctly, thereby decreasing incidence of noncompliance. Included are test for visual acuity, hearing and manual dexterity. In addition, an assessment of the patient's cognitive status will determine the type and amount of instruction appropriate for the older adult.

Treatment and Management

Many interventions lessen the incidence of polypharmacy in the elderly population. Health care professionals need to have a working knowledge of the pharmacokinetics of aging, drug-drug interactions and drug-disease interactions. Each new medication should be introduced using the "start low, go slow" principle, namely, starting at the lowest dosage and titrating upward in small increments until desired effect is achieved. Giving consideration to the altered risk-benefit ratio that exists for medications especially with regard to the old-old population is essential. Refills of medications should be closely monitored, especially PRN medications. Finally, non-pharmacological interventions should be encouraged whenever possible, especially for inducing sleep and reducing anxiety.

Education of the older adult regarding medications plays a critical part in fostering compliance and lessening occurrences of polypharmancy. The health care provider should keep the prescribed medication regimen as simple as possible. Verbal and written instructions should be provided for each prescribed medication. Written instructions should be designed to accommodate the older adult's decreased visual acuity. Encouraging the older adult to adopt a system for self administration of medications utilizing reminder aids e.g. clocks, calendars, and compartmentalized medication containers is valuable to foster compliance and lessen incidences of polypharmacy.

POLYPHARMACY ASSESSMENT

This checklist is designed to evaluate a patient's medication regimen in order to enhance compliance and to minimize the opportunity for the development of complications.

1. How many prescribed medications does the patient take?
2. How many nonprescription medications does the patient take?
3. What is the total number of medications taken by this patient?

If this total is 3 or more, then the patient is at risk for the complications of polypharmacy.

Circle "Yes" or "No" for the following:

Regarding the patient's medication regimen:

Y N – Have potential drug interactions been considered?
Y N – Has the medication been prescribed in the lowest effective dose?
Y N – Has the medication been adjusted for the patient's current rate of renal clearance?
Y N – Has the medication been adjusted for impaired hepatic function?
Y N – Have appropriate serum medication levels been monitored?
Y N – Are the medications prescribed on the simplest dosing regimen possible?
Y N – Are the patient's medications prescribed for the most appropriate route?
Y N – Are the medication directions in the appropriate language; are the labels in large print; are non-child resistant containers used?

Do the patients or their caregiver understand:

Y N – the name of the medication
Y N – the purpose of the medication
Y N – the dosage of the medication
Y N – the frequency of administration of the medication
Y N – the timing of administration of the medication
Y N – the relation to meals for the administration of the medications
Y N – the route of administration
Y N – the adverse reactions or side effects of which they should be aware
Y N – which medications may be crushed or chewed
Y N – has cost been considered in the prescription of the medications

In order to further enhance compliance:

Y N – have written and/or verbal instructions been supplied?
Y N – has a medication calendar been constructed?
Y N – has a packaging calendar (Medi-set) been considered?

If "N" is the circled response to any of the above questions, then consider consultation with the Pharmacy staff, the Nursing staff, and the caregivers in order to resolve the problems and minimize the risk to the patient.

Completed by _____

PREOPERATIVE ASSESSMENT

PREOPERATIVE ASSESSMENT OF THE GERIATRIC PATIENT

Significance

Preoperative assessment in the geriatric patient is important not only because seniors have higher rates of surgery, but especially because their rates of complications and mortality after surgery are significantly higher. Geriatric patients account for 75% of all postoperative deaths.

Etiology

The higher morbidity and mortality rates after surgery in the geriatric patient are due to the effects of aging on organ systems, the presence of multiple concurrent chronic illnesses which affect multiple organ systems, and the interactions between aging and diseases on the reserve potential of organ systems after a stress such as surgery. In addition, the fact that geriatric patients may appropriately require multiple medications for their chronic illnesses which may affect both organ system function and the response to injury and recovery.

All of these factors make the preoperative assessment of the older patient more important to perform, yet more difficult. The task is further complicated by another well known geriatric principle; that heterogeneity increases with age, so that each person must be evaluated as an individual, and no simple generalities or guidelines can be given for the individual patient for preoperative assessment. Along these lines, it should be carefully noted that age alone is a relatively poor predictor of surgical outcome when compared to other factors such as comorbid disease, severity of illness, functional status and others. This is important in the risk-benefit decisions regarding whether an individual should receive surgery. The increasing life expectancy of older adults also alters the equation in terms of the increasing number of years of functional life which may be saved by surgery in an individual.

Assessment

Older patients should have a general status assessment. This may include scales such as the American Society of Anesthesiology Physical Status Scale

Group	
Class I	healthy persons under age 80
Class II	healthy persons over age 80 with mild systemic disease
Class III	patients (regardless of age) with severe systemic disease (not incapacitating)
Class IV	patients with an incapacitating systemic disease that is a constant threat to life
Class V	patients who are moribund and not expected to live, with or without surgery

This scale is useful, and has predictive validity. Although it employs age as a risk factor, age is not a crucial risk factor in predicting postoperative outcomes; studies show that other factors are more important than age in predicting surgical outcomes employing this scale.

What are these other preoperative factors which predict postoperative outcomes? Functional status, nutritional status, and neuropsychological status (particularly dementia) are strong predictors of surgical outcome. Postoperative delirium is also a good predictor of surgical outcomes. In addition, organ specific diseases impact on surgical outcomes, primarily cardio-vascular disease, pulmonary disease, and renal disease. In particular, pre-existant ischemic heart disease or congestive heart failure predicts cardiac complications postoperatively. These factors are summarized in a "modified multifactorial index."

PREOPERATIVE ASSESSMENT

The purpose of this worksheet is to assist the team in the readying of the geriatric patient for surgical procedures.

A. Preoperative Studies

 Y N Complete blood count
 Y N Type and Hold/ Cross
 Y N Electrolytes
 Y N Urinalysis
 Y N Protime/Partial thromboplastin
 Y N Liver function tests
 Y N Chest X-ray
 Y N Electrocardiogram
 Y N Drug levels
 Y N Other

B. Preoperative Procedures

 Y N Consent form signed
 Y N Family members informed
 Y N Allergy list updated
 Y N Medication regimen modified
 Y N Preoperative note written

C. Specific Considerations

 Y N 1. Have the patient and/or caregiver been instructed in the use of equipment (such as spirometry) that will be used postoperatively?

 Y N 2. Does the patient have a pulmonary history such that pulmonary function tests or arterial blood gases should be checked?

 Y N 3. Does the patient have a baseline MiniMental State Examination and Activities of Daily Living score?

 Y N 4. Have the patient's preoperative and postoperative nutritional needs been assessed?

 Y N 5. Is the patient's immunocompetence status known?

 Y N 6. Is the patient at risk for the formation of a deep vein thrombosis or should anti-coagulation therapy be considered for the patient?

 Y N 7. Does the patient require antibiotic prophylaxis?

 Y N 8. Has the patient's Cardiac Risk Index been calculated? (see separate sheet)

 Y N 9. Are the patient's advanced directives documented?

Completed by _____

PREOPERATIVE RISK ASSESSMENT

CARDIAC RISK INDEX★

Circle the appropriate point totals

5	1.	Age greater than 70
10	2.	Myocardial infarction within the past six months
11	3.	Presence of S3 or gallop on cardiac exam
3	4.	"Significant" valvular aortic stenosis
7	5.	Rhythm other than sinus or presence of PACs on ECG
7	6.	More than 5 PVC's/min at any time prior to surgery
	7.	pO_2 less than 60 or pCO_2 greater than 50
3	8.	K+ less than 3.0 or HCO_3 less than 20 mEq/L
	9.	BUN greater than 50 or Creatinine greater than 3 mg/dL
	10.	Abnormal SGOT
	11.	Chronic liver disease
	12.	Bedridden due to non-cardiac cause
3	13.	Intraperitoneal, intrathoracic, or aortic surgery
4	14.	Emergency surgery

———————

TOTAL (53= maximum)

Class	Points	% Risk Cardiac Complication
I	0–5	1 %
II	6–12	7 %
II	13–25	14 %
IV	>25	78 %

Completed by _____

★ Adapted from Goldman L., Caldera D.L., Nussbaum S.R. *et al.*, Multifactorial index of cardiac risk in noncardiac surgical procedures. *N. Engl. J. Med.* 1977; **297**: 845-850.

Modified Multifactorial Index*	Points
Coronary artery disease	
Myocardial infarction within 6 months	10
Myocardial infarction more than 6 months	5
Canadian Cardiovascular Society angina	
Class III: walking 1–2 level blocks or 1 flight of stairs	10
Class IV: with any activity	20
Unstable angina within 6 months	10
Alveolar pulmonary edema	
within one week	10
ever	5
Valvular disease	20
Arrhythmias	
rhythm other than sinus or sinus plus atrial premature beats on last preoperative electrocardiogram	5
More than five premature ventricular contractions at any time prior to surgery	5
Poor general medical status (pO_2 <60 mmHg, pCO_2 >50 mmHg, K< 3.0 mEq/l, HCO_3 <20 mEq/l, BUN > 50 mEq/l, creatinine > 3.0 mg/dl, abnormal SGOT, signs of chronic liver disease, bedridden from noncardiac causes)	5
Age over 70	5
Emergency operation	10
Total score	

Risk class scoring:	
Class I	0–15
Class II (63% of all cardiac complications occured in patients with scores above 16)	15–30
Class III	>30

From: Detsky, A.S., Abrams, H.B., McLaughlin, J.R., Drucker, D.J., Sasson, Z., Johnson, N, Scott, J.G., Forbath, N., Hilliard, J.R. Predicting cardiac complications in patients undergoing non-cardiac surgery. *J. Gen. Intern. Med.* 1986; **1**: 211-219.

PRESSURE ULCERS

PRESSURE ULCERS IN OLDER ADULTS: PREVENTION AND TREATMENT

Significance of Problem

Pressure ulcers are painful, increase risk of infection, prolong hospitalization and increase mortality. Prevalence of pressure ulcers among patients in acute care settings is approximately 10 percent; among patients in skilled care and other nursing facilities as high as 23 percent. Estimated additional costs of medical and nursing care to treat pressure ulcer condition in one patient is up to $10,000.

Etiology

Pressure, as minimal as 60 mm Hg, to a body surface for 1-2 hours initiates the process of skin breakdown. Shear, friction, moisture and chemical irritants exacerbate the process. Older adults are at high risk for the development of pressure ulcers especially during hospitalization, but also while residing in nursing homes and living in the community. Factors which contribute to this risk include: increased age, immobility, incontinence, malnutrition and chronic illnesses such as diabetes and renal failure.

Prevention

Pressure ulcers are preventable. Prevention is accomplished by early identification of individuals at risk and implementation of interventions to reduce or eliminate these risks. Key elements of assessment to include are nutritional status, assessment for impediments to mobility, medication review especially for drugs increasing somnolence, and identification of causes of urinary and fecal incontinence. Concurrently, strategies must be in place to avoid direct pressure to bony prominences, as well as direct contact of two body surfaces.

Turning and positioning every 2 hours with the use of pillows for support is essential. Alternating pressure mattresses, foam wedges and pads facilitate pressure reduction. An overbed trapeze affords bed ridden patients a greater degree of mobility. The use of doughnuts, sheepskin pads and egg crates is discouraged because they relieve only surface pressure while providing a false sense of security.

Shear force results when friction between skin and a stationary surface holds the soft tissue in place while gravity pulls the axial skeleton down. Discourage the bed or chair bound patient from sitting with head elevated more than 30 degrees except for short periods of time.

Utilize moisture absorbent underpads or briefs to reduce exposure to moisture from urine and perspiration. Moisture softens the skin and increases risk of pressure ulcers.

Systematic skin inspection should occur on a daily basis with particular attention to bony prominences. Because erythema may not always be easily visualized, inspection should be accompanied by palpation for increased temperature and areas of induration. Cleansing of skin should occur with use of warm water and minimal friction. Moisturizers help to alleviate dry skin. Bony prominences should not be massaged.

Educate all care providers regarding preventive strategies.

Treatment and Management

Pressure ulcers occur most commonly on sacrum, hips, buttock, heels and/or lateral malleoli. Staging techniques are designed to identify the degree of tissue involvement. Staging is illustrated on the following table.

Stage	Characteristics	Treatment
I	non-blanchable erythema of intact skin	Avoid massage and pressure to involved area. Implement all relevant preventive measures. Film or hydrocolloid dressing may be needed based on location of ulcer. Continue to assess for risk factors.
II	partial thickness skin loss with epidermal involvement (may appear as abrasion, blister or shallow crater).	Treatments as outlined above with addition of petroleum gauze or semipermeable dressing to prevent dryness and protect healthy tissue
III	full thickness skin loss into subcutaneous tissue	Surgical or chemical debridement of necrotic tissue; cleanse wound with normal saline or whirlpool therapy; dress wound to ensure that ulcer tissue is kept moist while surrounding tissues are kept dry. Hydrocolloid dressings may be utilized. Consider use of specialized beds (low air loss or air-fluidized). Treat infection if present. Continue to assess for risk factors
IV	full thickness skin loss with extension beyond the deep fascia and involvement of muscle, bone, tendon or joint space	Treatment as outlined above. Wound packing may be needed based on the depth of wound. Continue to assess for risk factors.

Documentation during the course of treatment should include specifics about the size, location, stage of wound, presence of odor and purulent drainage and condition of surrounding tissues.

Pressure ulcers are usually colonized with multiple bacteria. Wound cultures are necessary in the presence of elevated temperature, purulent exudate and inflammation of surrounding tissues.

Utilize the multidisciplinary team approach to care for patients with pressure ulcers. Key functions of the nurse include monitoring of skin condition and educating patient and family member regarding strategies to prevent or lessen skin breakdown. Physical therapy will help to establish a program to address issues regarding mobility and conditioning. A nutritional consult will insure optimum nutritional support. Social services need to be incorporated into the plan of care for the community dwelling patient with pressure ulcers to facilitate the addition of services to assist in the completion of instrumental activities of daily living.

PRESSURE ULCER RISK ASSESSMENT*

The purpose of this tool is to identify those individuals who will be at risk for developing decubitus ulcers so that preventive measures may be instituted in a timely manner.

		Score
A.	**GENERAL PHYSICAL CONDITION**	
	1. Good (minor medical problems)	0
	2. Fair (major, but stable, medical problems)	1
	3. Poor (serious or unstable problems)	2
B.	**LEVEL OF CONSCIOUSNESS**	
	1. Alert (responds readily to verbal stimuli)	0
	2. Lethargic (responds slowly to verbal stimuli)	1
	3. Semi-comatose (responds to painful stimuli)	2
	4. Comatose (no response to stimuli)	3
C.	**ACTIVITY**	
	1. Ambulates without assistance	0
	2. Ambulates with assistance	2
	3. Chairbound	4
	4. Bedbound	6
D.	**EXTREMITY MOBILITY**	
	1. Full activity range	0
	2. Restricted movement	2
	3. Moves only with assistance	4
	4. Immobile	6
E.	**INCONTINENCE, BOWEL OR BLADDER**	
	1. None	0
	2. Occasionally (<2 episodes per 24 hours)	2
	3. Common (>2 episodes per 24 hours)	4
	4. Total	6
F.	**NUTRITION**	
	1. Good (consumes >50 % of meals)	0
	2. Fair (consumes 25-50% of meals)	1
	3. Poor (consumes <25% of meals)	2

TOTAL SCORE

ASSESSMENT :   AT RISK _____

If score is 8 or greater, notify the Nursing Staff of risk and necessary preventive measures

Completed by _____

* Adapted from Norton D. Calculating the risk: reflections on the Norton scale. *Decubitus.* 1989; **2**: 24-31.

SENSORY IMPAIRMENT ASSESSMENT

SENSORY IMPAIRMENT ASSESSMENTS

ASSESSMENT FOR HEARING LOSS IN THE OLDER ADULT

Significance of Problem

Alterations in the ability to hear begin in mid-life. It is estimated that as many as 40% of persons over the age of 65 experience some degree of hearing loss. Hearing impairment dramatically impacts on the quality of life of older adults, creating social isolation, depression and in some cases even paranoia. In addition, loss of hearing affects the safety of the older adult by inhibiting the individual's ability to respond to emergency situations and/or comprehend medical instructions. These inabilities often require the individual to relinquish independent living and relocate to a more supervised environment.

Etiology

Presbycusis, age related hearing loss, causes atrophy of the Organ of Corti, loss in numbers of auditory receptors, vascular changes and stiffening of the basilar membranes.

Other factors which place the older adult at risk for hearing impairment include:
*   excessive exposure to environmental noises
*   heredity
*   impacted cerumen
*   trauma
*   vascular, neurologic and infectious disease states
*   medications producing ototoxicity—aminoglycosides, antibiotics, salicylates, quinine.

Diagnosis

Medical History

Embarrassment, denial and lack of knowledge about treatment modalities contribute to the patient's reluctance to report hearing impairment to the primary care provider. Therefore, a specific direct question by the interviewer, such as "Have you noticed that you have to turn the TV up louder lately?", may be needed. Input from a family member may also contribute meaningful information about the extent of hearing impairment. Symptom analysis should include questions regarding onset, duration and progression of hearing impairment, unilateral or bilateral involvement, as well as presence of associated symptoms such as tinnitus or feeling of fullness in the ear.

Detailed past medical history should be obtained, as well as occupational history.

Record of current prescription and over-the-counter medication use is essential.

Inquire about the manner in which the ear is cleansed as part of daily personal hygiene routine. Finally, the impact hearing loss has had on the individual's ability to carry out daily activities is a relevant component of the medical history.

Physical Exam

Observe body language for indication of hearing impairment e.g. leaning forward, puzzled facial expression. Examine ear for presence of infection and impacted cerumen. Perform whispered voice, Weber and Rinné tests.

Diagnostic Testing

Individuals with acute hearing loss should be referred to an otolaryngologist for further evaluation. Referral to an audiologist for comprehensive audiometric studies is appropriate for individuals with chronic hearing loss.

Treatment and Management

If impacted cerumen is obvious on physical exam and patient has no history of prior perforation of tympanic membrane, gentle removal of cerumen can be attempted utilizing a cerumen spoon. Use of a cerumen softening agent, such as a hydrogen peroxide solution, should be advised to avoid further cerumen accumulations.

Educate family members about effective communication techniques. These include eliminating background noises, facing the listener, speaking slowly and clearly with avoidance of shouting.

Educate patient about availability of adaptive devices for telephone and television, amplification systems, and self help groups for hearing impaired.

SENSORY IMPAIRMENT ASSESSMENTS

Hearing Handicap Inventory for the Elderly-Screening Version (HHIE-S)	Score
Does a hearing problem cause you to feel embarassed when you meet new people?	
Does a hearing problem cause you to feel frustrated when talking to members of your family?	
Do you have difficulty hearing when someone speaks in a whisper?	
Do you feel handicapped by a hearing problem?	
Does a hearing problem cause you difficulty when visiting friends, relatives or neighbors?	
Does a hearing problem cause you to attend religious services less often than you would like?	
Does a hearing problem cause you to have arguments with your family?	
Does a hearing problem cause you difficulty when listening to television or radio?	
Do you feel that any difficulty with your hearing limits hampers your personal or social life?	
Does a hearing problem cause you difficulty when in a restaurant with relatives or friends?	
Total score:	

HEARING ASSESSMENT

Scoring: "no" response = 0; "sometimes" = 2; "yes" =4; maximum score = 40.
Scores between 10-24 indicate some hearing impairment; scores above 24 indicate significant hearing problems.

On examination:

	Yes/No
A. Abnormal external ear	
B. Abnormal otoscopic exam	
C. Abnormal brief audiometry	
D. Abnormal "whisper" test	
E. Does the patient wear a hearing aid? If so, is it functioning properly?	
F. Other (specify):	

Previous studies indicate that persons require referral to otolaryngology or audiology for further evaluation if they either 1) have an abnormal audioscopic examination and a score greater than 8 on the HHIE-S; or 2) score greater than 24 on the HHIE-S

Completed by _____

Adapted from: Lichenstein, M.J., Bess F.H., Logan, S.A. Validation of screening tools for identifying hearing impaired elderly in primary care. *J. Amer. Med. Assoc.* 1988; **259**: 2875-2878.

ASSESSING VISION IN THE OLDER ADULT

Significance of Problem

A decline in visual acuity begins at around age 50. Visual loss is experienced by about twenty percent of the older adult population and impacts on the quality of life of these individuals. Driving, an activity which contributes to one's ability to socialize and remain independent, must frequently be curtailed because of loss of vision. Instrumental activities of daily living, such as shopping, banking, meal preparation and self administration of medications may also be impaired by a decline in vision. Poor vision is a contributing factor to falls in the elderly, and may lead to social withdrawal and depression.

Etiology

Presbyopia, loss of accommodation, is the primary visual change experienced by older adults and results from physiological changes in the lens. Other age related changes include an increased sensitivity to glare, decreased depth perception, diminished visual fields, increased time to adapt to darkness and impaired color discrimination.

Macular degeneration, glaucoma, cataracts and diabetic retinopathy can result in progressive visual loss.

Diagnosis

Medical History

The older adult may not be aware of gradual loss of vision or may consider it a normal process of aging and, as a result, not report it to the health care provider. A direct question, such as "Are you having any difficulty reading the newspaper or watching television?' is helpful. Specific questions regarding glare sensitivity, difficulty with night driving, loss of visual fields, tearing, eye irritation, eye pain and diplopia are relevant.

Inquire about the frequency and etiology of falls.

Review current medication use.

Obtain information about frequency of eye exam by ophthalmologist.

Detailed medical history should be obtained with emphasis on diabetes, hypertension and cerebrovascular disease.

Physical Exam

Test for visual acuity with Snellen or Jaeger eye chart. As an alternative have the patient read a few lines from headline and regular newsprint. Examine the external structures of the eye with particular attention to the presence of ectropion (lower lid margin not in contact with eyeball) or entropion (inversion of a relaxed lid). Assess visual fields. Perform fundoscopic exam.

Observation of the patient's gait will also assist in evaluation of visual acuity.

Treatment and Management

History and physical findings will determine treatment options. Recent, sudden vision loss warrants prompt referral to an ophthalmologist. Asymptomatic patients with negative physical findings should receive a recommendation for annual exam by ophthalmologist.

Educate the patient about interventions to lessen impact of age related visual changes. These strategies include increasing amount of illumination, decreasing glare and use of night lights.

A home evaluation by an occupational therapist can result in the introduction of low vision aids to facilitate use of telephone, administration of medications and operation of household appliances.

Referral to a self help group will serve to lessen the individual's anxiety while increasing knowledge about other resources to broaden opportunities for communication.

SENSORY IMPAIRMENT ASSESSMENTS

VISION ASSESSMENT

	Yes	No
1. Examination by Ophthamologist greater than one year ago?		
2. Complaints of visual disturbances or changes?		
3. Examination		
A. Abnormal acuity:		
B. Abnormal visual fields:		
C. Abnormal fundus:		
D. Abnormal external eye:		
E. Other (specify):		

"YES" to any item, contact Ophthalmology.

Completed by _____

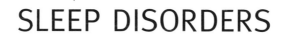

SLEEP DISORDERS

SLEEP DISORDERS

Significance

Sleep disorders are common in the elderly and the primary care provider will often have patients with complaints of sleep disturbances. About 20-40% of people in their 70s may complain of sleep disturbances which may be more common in men.

Age-related changes in the amount and pattern of sleep with normal aging have been described. Older persons experience a reduction in slow-wave, or stage 4, sleep, increased nighttime wakefulness and increased fragmentation of sleep by periods of wakefulness. There are less significant changes in REM sleep and total nighttime sleep. Older persons are also more easily aroused from sleep. With advanced age, changes in circadian sleep-wake rhythms may occur, with increased nighttime wakefulness and more daytime fatigue and napping.

However, as with other geriatric disorders in old age, there is also great inter-individual variability, and the effects of normal aging in an individual must be distinguished from potentially reversible causes of sleep disorders, as well as diseases which may causes sleep disorders.

Causes of Sleep Disorders

Sleep disorders may be categorized into primary and secondary causes. A variety of medical illnesses may cause sleep disorders. The causes of sleep disorders have been categorized by the International Classification of Diseases (ICD-9). The major categories are:

I.   Dyssomnias
    A. **Intrinsic sleep disorders:** examples include obstructive sleep apnea, periodic limb movement disorder, narcolepsy.
    B. **Extrinsic sleep disorders:** examples include inadequate sleep hygiene, adjustment sleep disorder, stimulant or alcohol dependent sleep disorder, environmental problems including excess noise, lighting and high or low room temperatures
    C. **Circadian rhythm sleep disorders:** examples include time-zone change syndrome, irregular sleep-wake pattern, delay/advanced sleep phase syndrome
II. Parasomnias
    A. **Arousal disorders**: including confusional arousal, sleepwalking
III. Sleep disorders associated with medical or psychiatric disorders
    A. **Neuropsychiatric disorders**: including dementia, mood disorders, alcoholism
    B. **Neurological disorders:** including Parkinsonism
    C. **Medical disorders:** including nocturnal angina, gastroesophageal reflux, COPD, chronic pain syndromes, incontinence and medications.

Assessment

Sleep disorders can generally be diagnosed and managed by the primary care practitioner without the use of sophisticated technology. Patients should be asked about their sleep patterns and a history taken to investigate the possible causes of sleep problems. Sleep pattern questions should include time to fall asleep, duration of sleep, time, number and duration of wakenings, daytime sleep patterns including naps. Information from sleep partners is often useful in evaluating the patient, and also gives a determination of the relative impact of the sleep disturbance on the partner.

A medical history may reveal underlying medical causes, including medications, foods and beverages which frequently cause sleep disturbances in the elderly.

An environmental history may reveal factors, such as excessive noise, lighting, or room temperatures which impair sleep.

A history of snoring and its characterization is important in evaluating apneas. If the history seems unreliable, or more careful information is required, then a 24 hour sleep log is useful to determine actual sleep-wake cycles. These logs can be kept by patients themselves, but are generally more accurately kept by sleep partners or caregivers. Obviously, this is crucial in the demented patient.

Referral to the sleep laboratory is generally only required in cases of obstructive sleep apnea or periodic limb movement disorder, especially to determine the severity and risk of the disorder.

Management and Treatment

Sleep disturbances not only impair quality of life, but they also lead to morbidity and mortality through daytime accidents, impaired quality of life for caregivers, and in the case of apneas increased risk of medical illnesses. Good sleep hygiene is crucial to encouraging sleep without medications. Reassurance is often all that is needed in an elderly patient who is experiencing changes associated with normal aging.

Attention to an appropriate mattress free of impediments, a supportive pillow, appropriate lighting, noise levels, and temperature are all important. Eliminate daytime napping, insure the patient obtains adequate daytime exposure to sunlight, and encourage exercise. Avoid caffeine, drink hot milk (contains tryptophan) before bedtime, avoid alcohol, reduce nocturnal consumption of liquids if the patient is incontinent and encourage the practice of a bedtime ritual such as reading or music. Caregivers or sleep partners of snoring sleepers can use earplugs or schemes to obtain adequate sleep.

Medications such as hypnotics should be avoided, particularly in patients with obstructive sleep apnea and COPD where they are contraindicated. In cases where immediate correction of altered sleep patterns is needed to relieve suffering, only short acting hypnotics should be employed, and only for brief (up to one-two weeks) periods. The safety and efficacy of melatonin has not been established in the elderly and cannot be recommended at this time.

Patients with obstructive sleep apnea should be referred for further evaluation and consideration of continuous positive airway pressure at night.

SLEEP DISORDERS ASSESSMENT

The purpose of this tool is to assist the examiner in the evaluation and treatment of sleep disorders

CIRCLE THE APPROPRIATE RESPONSE

Y N 1.   Does the sleep disorder interfere with daytime activities?
Y N 2.   Does the patient have an unusually early or late time for retiring to bed?
          If so, what is it?
Y N 3.   Does the patient have an unusually early or late time for rising?
          If so, what is it?
Y N 4.   Does it take a long time for the patient to fall asleep?
          If so, how long does it usually take?
Y N 5.   Does the patient spend the majority of their time in bed?
Y N 6.   Does the patient awaken in the middle of the night?
          If so, how often does this occur?
          Why do the awakenings occur?
Y N   a. need to use the bathroom
Y N   b. nightmares
Y N   c. worrying about something
Y N   d. loss of breath
Y N   e. pain
Y N   f. loud shoring
Y N   g. leg twitching
Y N   h. other
Y N 7.   Does the patient wander at night?
Y N 8.   During the day, does the patient:
Y N   a. take frequent naps
Y N   b. take few, long naps
Y N   c. have any exercise periods
Y N 9.   At night does the spouse or caretaker note:
Y N   a. loud snoring
Y N   b. periods of apnea
Y N   c. restless legs
Y N   d. leg jerks
Y N 10.   Does the patients location of sleep have:
Y N   a. adequate temperature regulation
Y N   b. adequate sound control
Y N   c. appropriate lighting
Y N 11.   Is the bed used for activities other than sleep or sexual activities?
Y N 12.   Are there medical conditions that may interfere with sleep?
          If so, what are they?

Y N 13. Does the patient consume or use any of the following?
If so, state what time of the day they are consumed.
Y N   a. coffee
Y N   b. tea
Y N   c. sodas
Y N   d. tobacco
Y N   e. alcohol
Y N   f. OTC sleeping aids
Y N   g. prescribed sleeping medications (for how long?)
Y N   h. diuretics
Y N   i. sympathomimetics
Y N 14. Has depression been ruled out?
Y N 15. Has dementia been ruled out?

THE PROBABLE CAUSE OF THE PATIENT'S SLEEP DISORDER IS:

Dyssomnias
> **Intrinsic sleep disorders:**
>> obstructive sleep apnea
>> periodic limb movement disorder
>> narcolepsy
>
> **Extrinsic sleep disorders:** examples include inadequate sleep hygiene, adjustment sleep disorder, stimulant or alcohol dependent sleep disorder, environmental problems including excess noise, lighting and high or low room temperatures
> **Circadian rhythm sleep disorders:** examples include time-zone change syndrome, irregular sleep-wake pattern, delay/advanced sleep phase syndrome

Parasomnias
> **Arousal disorders**: including confusional arousal, sleepwalking

Sleep disorders associated with medical or psychiatric disorders
> **Neuropsychiatric disorders:** including dementia, mood disorders, alcoholism
> **Neurological disorders:** including Parkinsonism
> **Medical disorders**: including nocturnal angina, gastroesophageal reflux, COPD, chronic pain syndromes, incontinence and medications.

Consider consultation with Sleep Disorders specialist in patients with obstructive sleep apnea, and difficult to diagnose patients in whom the sleep disorder is an important cause of functional impairment

Completed by _____

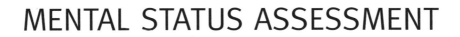

MENTAL STATUS ASSESSMENT

COGNITIVE IMPAIRMENT IN THE ELDERLY

Significance

The three leading causes of cognitive impairment in the elderly are dementia, depression and delirium, respectively. Dementia affects approximately 5% of all individuals over the age of 65 years, and up to 25-45% of individuals over the age of 80 years, and is the leading cause of disability in the "old-old". Depression is also a common illness in the elderly, also affecting up to 5% of individuals over the age 65, although estimates vary widely. Delirium affects primarily hospitalized patients, but may be a cause of cognitive impairment in community dwelling elderly who have suffered a relatively acute change in mental status.

Assessment

One of the first steps in the evaluation of the patient with cognitive complaints is the documentation of cognitive impairment employing validated assessment instruments. That is, does the patient truly have cognitive impairment?

A valuable screening tool for the documentation of cognitive impairment is the MiniMental State Examination. This tool assesses the cognitive status of an elderly individual and can determine the presence of cognitive impairment with considerable reliability. It is a brief, validated screening instrument for the presence of cognitive impairment. It does not, however, provide the cause of the cognitive impairment, and has certain limitations. For example, the tool has somewhat limited sensitivity in patients with very mild cognitive impairment. For these patients, more careful neuropsychological testing is required, particularly when the history provided by either the patient or their caregivers indicates a clear change in cognitive function, and/or the functional activities of daily living.

If a patient has documented cognitive impairment, then the cause of the cognitive impairment must be determined.

If the duration of the cognitive impairment is relatively short (less than six weeks), then the diagnosis of delirium must be considered. Delirium is a medical diagnosis characterized by attentional deficits, with a waxing and waning of confusion and state of consciousness. A medical evaluation for causes of delirium must be performed, particularly since delirium may be the first sign of a medical illness. There are validated instruments for the detection and diagnosis of delirium in the acute setting.

If delirium has been eliminated as a possibility, then chronic causes of cognitive impairment in the elderly must be considered. These include primarily dementia and depression.

The first step in making a diagnosis of dementia is the characterization of the nature of cognitive impairment. Generally, a patient with dementia will present with a history of chronic, progressive cognitive and functional loss, with complaints of confusion, disorientation, memory loss, difficulty with communication and other cognitive symptoms. Often, a patient's family member or caregiver is the first to note such problems, although sometimes the patient themselves will be the primary source of complaint. The clinician's role is to determine the specific nature of the cognitive deficits, their duration, and the manner in which such deficits impair daily function. The DSM IV criteria for the diagnosis of dementia are useful in structuring the clinical and neuropsychological interview and in making a diagnosis of dementia.

Once a diagnosis of dementia is made according to standard criteria, then the cause of the dementia must be determined. Alzheimer's disease is the leading cause of dementia in this population. Other primary degenerative diseases may also cause dementia, including Lewy body disease, which has recently been recognized as more common than previously thought. The second most common group of causes of dementia are cerebrovascular disease, including multiinfarct dementia, lacunar dementia (or microvascular dementia), and other types of vascular dementia. In the very old, vascular dementia may be the leading cause of dementia. There are widely used scales for vascular dementia, particularly the Hachinski ischemic score.

In addition to these "primary" causes of dementia, there are also "secondary" or potentially reversible causes of dementia, including depression, B12 deficiency, thyroid disease, normal pressure hydrocephalus, and brain tumors. These secondary causes account for about 10% of all cases presenting with cognitive impairment in the ambulatory care setting. Depression with cognitive impairment is the most common cause of secondary cognitive impairment, and may be difficult to distinguish from dementia with depressive symptoms.

Depression should always be considered as a cause of cognitive impairment. A number of brief screening instruments are available with good sensitivity and specificity in the elderly. Generally, during the clinical interview, the patient with dementia will make considerable attempts at providing answers to questions, trying to prove their cognitive capacity, while the patient with depression may exhibit little motivation or attempt to answer questions by the clinician. Vegetative symptoms, such as changes in eating or sleeping habits, are more often characteristic of early depression than early dementia. Employing standardized criteria for depression helps to organize the diagnostic interview. However, it is often difficult to distinguish the patient with dementia and associated depressive symptoms from the patient with depression and concomitant cognitive impairment.

Management and Treatment

The management and treatment of dementia is complex and beyond the scope of this brief manual. There are some excellent texts for the management of dementia. Some brief elements of management are mentioned here. Most aspects of the management of dementia focus on maintaining functional capacity and a supportive environment. Although some medical treatments focused on cognitive enhancement are available, none of these treatments is known to prevent progressive cognitive decline at this time. Treatment of the comorbid emotional disorders commonly associated with dementia, such as agitation and depression, is generally warranted and worthwhile.

Education of family members and caregivers regarding disease progression and appropriate approaches to long term care of the demented patient is essential. Printed materials and participation in support groups can effectively supplement verbal instructions by the provider.

Advanced directives should be obtained early in the course of the illness while patients are still capable of understanding and providing accurate statements and judgements to express their wishes. Most of the ultimate comorbidities of dementia which lead to decline and death are related to functional impairment which eventually result in infections, such as malnutrition, aspiration, incontinence and immobility. Accidents are also a major cause of morbidity and mortality. Hospice care is often appropriate at the end stages of dementia.

Depressive symptoms and cognitive impairment often present simultaneously in the elderly. About 30% of individuals with early dementia have depressive symptoms, while mild cognitive impairment is common among elderly depressed individuals. Although it may be difficult to distinguish the patient with dementia and associated depressive symptoms from the patient with depression and concomitant cognitive impairment, in either case treating the patient for depression is of benefit. The patient with dementia may have improved mood, less dysphoria, and possibly some secondary benefit on cognition, although the fundamental, progressive cognitive dysfunction will continue. In the patient with depression, mood will improve and cognitive impairment may resolve. Thus, treatment may be of diagnostic value; mild cognitive impairment should dissipate in the successfully treated depressed patient, while cognitive impairment will persist in the patient with primary dementia.

Algorithm for the diagnostic evaluation of cognitive impairment in the elderly

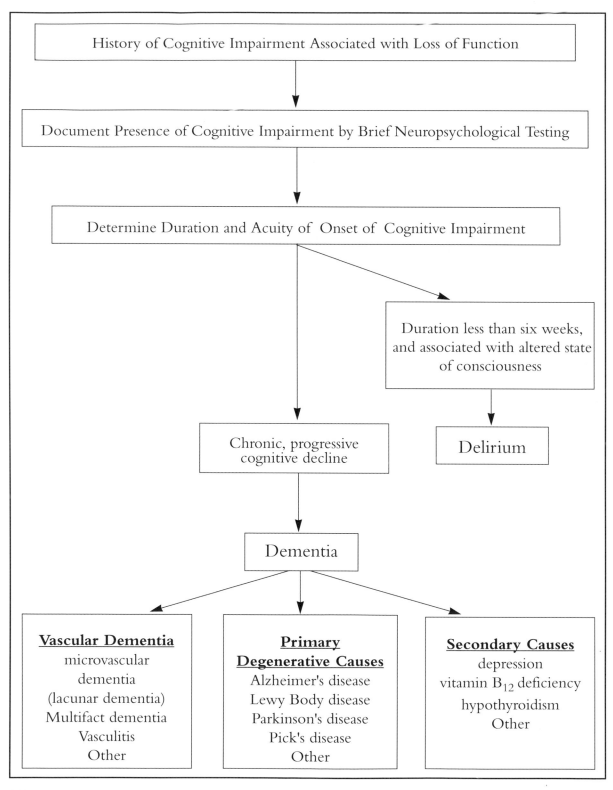

ASSESSING DEPRESSION IN THE OLDER ADULT

Significance of Problem

Depression is the most common mental health problem among older adults. Degrees of severity vary from mild cases of dysphoria occurring in about 10% of the older adult population to extreme cases with psychotic features and/or suicidal ideations affecting about 5% of the elderly. Depression in the older adult can lead to malnutrition, dehydration, falls, noncompliance with medical regimen and suicide. Suicide rates in our society are highest among elderly, white males.

Etiology

Many factors place an older adult at risk for depression:
- genetic predisposition
- prior history of depression
- sensory losses - especially diminished hearing and vision
- social losses of aging - loss of independence, death of friends and spouse, retirement
- chronic disease states - cerebrovascular disease, dementia, Parkinson's disease, cardio-vascular disease, COPD, alcoholism, hypothyroidism,
- medications such as antihypertensives, sedatives and analgesics

Diagnosis

Medical History

The older patient will frequently not self report feelings of sadness or depression. Sometimes, the elderly may view these depressive symptoms as "normal" part of aging, or not wish to be viewed as a burden by the clinician or family. As a result, the elderly often somatize depressed feelings and instead verbalize to the clinician physical complaints such as muscloskeletal symptoms, rapid heart rate and gastrointestinal complaints. In this way, depression frequently leads to increased and sometimes inappropriate health care utilization.

In the depressed patient, a review of symptoms may uncover complaints of insomnia, constipation, anorexia, unintentional weight loss, lethargy and apathy. Ask direct questions about feelings of sadness and hopelessness. If the patient does verbalize feelings of hopelessness, ask specific questions regarding suicidal ideations. An example of such a question is " Sometimes when people are sad, they have thoughts about harming themselves. Have you ever had thoughts like these?"

Obtain a detailed medication history including over-the-counter drug use as well as a comprehensive past medical history including history of prior depression. Psychosocial history should include family dynamics, caregiver support, recent losses and the patient's opportunities for socializing and meaningful activity.

Physical Exam

It may be difficult to distinguish clinical signs of depression from underlying comorbities. Particular attention should, however, be paid to the patient's general physical appearance, condition of clothing and personal hygiene, facial expression and eye contact.

In addition to a comprehensive physical, including neurologic exam, a functional assessment and specific validated assessments of cognitive function and depression will facilitate formulation of differential diagnoses.

Laboratory Tests

Laboratory tests to assist in the assessment of depression include complete blood count, blood chemistries, vitamin B12 and folate levels, thyroid, renal and liver function tests. Other diagnostic testing should be done based on patient's somatic complaints and physical findings.

Treatment and Management

Employ DSM IV Criteria for Major Depressive Episode to make the diagnosis of depression. History, physical findings, laboratory data will assist in determining potentially reversible causes and directed treatment modalities. Treatment of underlying acute and chronic medical conditions should be optimized and medication regimens adjusted as needed. Chronic pain and functional disability are often contributing factors to depression in the elderly.

The patient experiencing acute psychosis or suicidal ideations will require hospitalization in most cases. In severe cases, electroshock treatment may be appropriate and effective in the elderly. Outpatient care should include psychotherapy and antidepressant medication therapy for the depressed patient who is not a danger to himself.

In patient's with mild depression, social services are an important adjunct to counseling and antidepressant therapy. Social services can assist the patient with opportunities for socialization. Examples of such programs include volunteer organizations, senior centers, adult day care and "friendly visitors". Self help group participation may also be helpful for patients experiencing dysphoria. A social worker may also provide psychotherapy for elderly patients.

There are many stereotypes about mental health disease in our society. Patient and family education about the high prevalence of depression in older adults, the risks of suicide, the many causes and the fact that most depressed patients can be effectively treated is essential to foster acceptance of the diagnosis and compliance to the medical regimen.

AFFECTIVE DISORDERS ASSESSMENT

ASSESSMENT OF AFFECTIVE DISORDERS

YESAVAGE GERIATRIC DEPRESSION SCALE★

1. ARE YOU BASICALLY SATISFIED WITH YOUR LIFE? YES NO

2. HAVE YOU DROPPED MANY OF YOUR ACTIVITIES
AND INTERESTS? YES NO

3. DO YOU FEEL THAT YOUR LIFE IS EMPTY? YES NO

4. DO YOU OFTEN GET BORED? YES NO

5. ARE YOU HOPEFUL ABOUT THE FUTURE? YES NO

6. ARE YOU BOTHERED BY THOUGHTS YOU CAN'T
GET OUT OF YOUR HEAD? YES NO

7. ARE YOU IN GOOD SPIRITS MOST OF THE TIME? YES NO

8. ARE YOU AFRAID THAT SOMETHING BAD IS GOING
TO HAPPEN TO YOU? YES NO

9. DO YOU FEEL HAPPY MOST OF THE TIME? YES NO

10. DO YOU OFTEN FEEL HELPLESS? YES NO

11. DO YOU OFTEN GET RESTLESS AND FIDGETY? YES NO

12. DO YOU PREFER TO STAY AT HOME, RATHER THAN
GOING OUT AND DOING NEW THINGS? YES NO

13. DO YOU FREQUENTLY WORRY ABOUT THE FUTURE? YES NO

14. DO YOU FEEL YOU HAVE MORE PROBLEMS WITH
MEMORY THAN MOST? YES NO

15. DO YOU THINK IT IS WONDERFUL TO BE ALIVE NOW? YES NO

16. DO YOU OFTEN FEEL DOWNHEARTED AND BLUE? YES NO

17. DO YOU FEEL PRETTY WORTHLESS THE WAY YOU ARE NOW?   YES   NO

18. DO YOU WORRY A LOT ABOUT THE PAST?   YES   NO

19. DO YOU FIND LIFE VERY EXCITING?   YES   NO

20. IS IT HARD FOR YOU TO GET STARTED ON NEW PROJECTS?   YES   NO

21. DO YOU FEEL FULL OF ENERGY?   YES   NO

22. DO YOU FEEL THAT YOUR SITUATION IS HOPELESS?   YES   NO

23. DO YOU THINK THAT MOST PEOPLE ARE BETTER OFF THAN YOU ARE?   YES   NO

24. DO YOU FREQUENTLY GET UPSET OVER LITTLE THINGS?   YES   NO

25. DO YOU FREQUENTLY FEEL LIKE CRYING?   YES   NO

26. DO YOU HAVE TROUBLE CONCENTRATING?   YES   NO

27. DO YOU ENJOY GETTING UP IN THE MORNING?   YES   NO

28. DO YOU PREFER TO AVOID SOCIAL GATHERINGS?   YES   NO

29. IS IT EASY FOR YOU TO MAKE DECISIONS?   YES   NO

30. IS YOUR MIND AS CLEAR AS IT USED TO BE?   YES   NO

★ Adapted from Yesavage, J.A., Brink, T.L., Rose, T.L. *et al.* Development and validation of a geriatric depression screening scale: a preliminary report. *J. Psychiatr. Res.* 1983; **17**: 37-49.

ASSESSMENT OF AFFECTIVE DISORDERS

SCORESHEET FOR GERIATRIC DEPRESSION SCALE

1.	NO	Score 1 point for each of the
2.	YES	patient's answers that matches
3.	YES	this scoresheet
4.	YES	
5.	NO	Total all of the points
6.	YES	
7.	NO	
8.	YES	_____ TOTAL
9.	NO	
10.	YES	
11.	YES	
12.	YES	
13.	YES	
14.	YES	Scoring:
15.	NO	
16.	YES	0-9 Normal
17.	YES	
18.	YES	10-19 Mild depressive
19.	NO	
20.	YES	20-30 Severe depressive
21.	NO	
22.	YES	
23.	YES	
24.	YES	
25.	YES	
26.	YES	
27.	NO	
28.	YES	
29.	NO	
30.	NO	

Completed by _____

DSM IV Criteria for Major Depressive Episode

A. Five (or more) of the following symptoms have been present during the same 2-week period and represent a change from previous functioning; at least one of the symptoms is either (1) depressed mood or (2) loss of interest or pleasure.

Note: Do not include symptoms that are clearly due to a general medical condition, or mood-incongruent delusions or hallucinations.

(1) depressed mood most of the day, nearly every day, as indicated by either subjective report (e.g., feels sad or empty) or observation made by others (e.g., appears tearful).

(2) markedly diminished interest or pleasure in all, or almost all, activities most of the day, nearly every day (as indicated by either subjective account or observation made by others)

(3) significant weight loss when not dieting or weight gain (e.g., a change of more than 5% of body weight in a month), or decrease or increase in appetite nearly every day.

(4) insomnia or hypersomnia nearly every day

(5) psychomotor agitation or retardation nearly every day (observable by others, not merely subjective feelings of restlessness or being slowed down)

(6) fatigue or loss of energy nearly every day

(7) feelings of worthlessness or excessive or inappropriate guilt (which may be delusional) nearly every day (not merely self-reproach or guilt about being sick)

(8) diminished ability to think or concentrate, or indecisiveness, nearly every day (either by subjective account or as observed by others)

(9) recurrent thought of death (not just fear of dying), recurrent suicidal ideation without a specific plan, or a suicide attempt or a specific plan for committing suicide

B. The symptoms do not meet criteria for a Mixed Episode.

C. The symptoms cause clinically significant distress of impairment in social, occupational, or other important areas of functioning.

D. The symptoms are not due to the direct physiological effects of a substance (e.g., a drug of abuse, or a medication) or a general medical condition (e.g., hypothyroidism).

E. The symptoms are not better accounted for by bereavement, i.e., after the loss of a loved one, the symptoms persist for longer than 2 months or are characterized by marked functional impairment, morbid preoccupation with worthlessness, suicidal ideation, psychotic symptoms, or psychomotor retardation.

American Psychiatric Association Committee on Nomenclature and Statistics, *Diagnostic and Statistical Manual of Mental Disorders*, Washington, DC: American Psychiatric Association, 1994.

COGNITIVE ASSESSMENT

MINI-MENTAL STATE EXAM★

ORIENTATION:

time: date _____   month _____   year _____   season _____   day _____

current location: state _____   city _____   street _____   country _____   floor _____

REGISTRATION: dog _____   apple _____   table _____

ATTENTION & CALCULATION:

serial 7's: 93 ____   86 ____   79 ____   72 ____   65 ____

or: world: dlrow _____

RECALL: dog _____   apple _____   table _____

LANGUAGE: pencil _____   watch _____

"no ifs, ands, or buts" _____

Three step command: right hand _____   fold _____   on floor _____

MINI-MENTAL STATE EXAM (continued)

Read: **CLOSE YOUR EYES.**

Write a sentence: _____

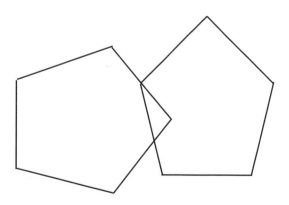

Score: (Maximum 30) _____   Examiner _____

Interpretation: If scores > 24, probably no cognitive impairment:; for scores 20-24, patients need further cognitive testing, unless educational/cultural/language effects are thought to play a role; scores less than 20 indicate cognitive impairment..

★Adapted from Folstein, M., Folstein, S., McHugh, P.R. Mini Mental State: a practical method for grading the cognitive state of patients for the clinician. *J. Psychiat. Res.* 1975; **12** 189-198.

DSM IV Diagnostic criteria for Dementia of the Alzheimer's Type

A. The development of multiple cognitive deficits manifested by both

   (1) memory impairment (impaired ability to learn new information or to recall previously learned information)

   (2) one (or more) of the following cognitive disturbances:

      (a) aphasia (language disturbance)

      (b) apraxia (impaired ability to carry out motor activities despite intact motor function)

      (c) agnosia (failure to recognize or identify objects despite intact sensory function)

      (d) disturbance in executive functioning (i.e., planning, organizing, sequencing, abstracting)

B. The cognitive deficits in Criteria A1 and A2 each cause significant impairment in social or occupational functioning and represent a significant decline from a previous level of functioning.

C. The course is characterized by gradual onset and continuing cognitive decline.

D. The cognitive deficits in Criteria A1 and A2 are not due to any of the following:

   (1) other central nervous system conditions that cause progressive deficits in memory and cognition (e.g., cerebrovascular disease, Parkinson's disease, Huntington's disease, subdural hematoma, normal-pressure hydrocephalus, brain tumor)

   (2) systemic conditions that are known to cause dementia (e.g., hypothyroidism, vitamin B_{12} or folic acid deficiency, niacin deficiency, hypercalcemia, neurosyphilis, HIV infection)

   (3) substance-induced conditions

E. The deficits do not occur exclusively during the course of a delirium.

F. The disturbance is not better accounted for by another Axis I disorder (e.g., Major Depressive Disorder, Schizophrenia).

Code based on type of onset and predominant features:

> **With Early Onset**: if onset is at age 65 years or below
> **290.11 With Delirium**: if delirium is superimposed on the dementia
> **290.12 With Delusions**: if delusions are the predominant feature
> **290.13 With Depressed Mood**: if depressed moods (including presentations that meet full symptom criteria for a Major Depressive Episode) is the predominant feature. A separate diagnosis of Mood Disorder Due to a General Medical Condition is not given.
> **290.10 Uncomplicated**: if none of the above predominates in the current clinical presentation

> **With Late Onset**: if onset is after 65 years
> **290.3 With Delirium**: if delirium is superimposed on the dementia
> **290.20 With Delusions:** if delusions are the predominant feature
> **290.21 With Depressed Mood:** if depressed moods (including presentations that meet full symptom criteria for a Major Depressive Episode) is the predominant feature. A separate diagnosis of Mood Disorder Due to a General Medical Condition is not given.
> **290.0 Uncomplicated**: if none of the above predominates in the current clinical presentation

Specify if:
With Behavioral Disturbance

Coding note: Also code 331.0 Alzheimer's disease on Axis III.

Criteria for Severity of Dementia:

Mild: Although work or social activities are significantly impaired, the capacity for independent living remains, with adequate personal hygiene and relatively intact judgement.

Moderate: independent living is hazardous and some degree of supervision is necessary.

Severe: activities of daily living are so impaired that continual supervision is required; (eg. unable to maintain minimal personal hygiene; largely incoherent or mute; the patient is completely dependent.)

American Psychiatric Association Committee on Nomenclature and Statistics. *Diagnostic and Statistical Manual of Mental Disorders.* Washington, DC: American Psychiatric Association, 1994.

COGNITIVE ASSESSMENT

HACHINSKI ISCHEMIC SCORE★

This scale was developed for the diagnosis of multi-infarct dementia.

	Score
1. Abrupt Onset	2
2. Stepwise deterioration	1
3. Fluctuating course	2
4. Nocturnal confusion	1
5. Relative preservation of personality	1
6. Depression	1
7. Somatic complaints	1
8. Emotional incontinence	1
9. History of hypertension	1
10. History of strokes	2
11. Evidence of associated atherosclerosis	1
12. Focal neurological symptoms	2
13. Focal neurological signs	2

A total score of 7 or greater suggests a vascular component of dementia.

★ Adapted from: Hachinski V.C. Vascular dementia: a radical redefinition. *Dementia.* 1994; **5**: 130.

LOEB'S MODIFIED ISCHEMIC SCORE★

This scale was developed as a modification of the Hachinski scale for the diagnosis of multi-infarct or vascular dementia.

Circle the appropriate score for each item

1. Abrupt onset	2
2. History of stroke	1
3. Focal symptoms	2
4. Focal signs	2
5. CT-low density areas	
isolated	2
multiple	3

(maximum score is 9–10) _____ TOTAL

0–2 consistent with SDAT

3–4 is equivocal

5–10 consistent with MID

Completed by _____

★ Adapted from: Loeb, C., Gandolfo, C. Diagnostic evaluation of degenerative and vascular dementia. *Stroke*. 1983; **14**: 399.

DSMIV Diagnostic criteria for Vascular Dementia

A. The development of multiple cognitive deficits manifested by both

    (1) memory impairment (impaired ability to learn new information or to recall previously learned information)

    (2) one (or more) of the following cognitive disturbances:

        (a) aphasia (language disturbance)

        (b) apraxia (impaired ability to carry out motor activities despite intact motor function)

        (c) agnosia (failure to recognize or identify objects despite intact sensory function)

        (d) disturbance in executive functioning (i.e., planning, organizing, sequencing, abstracting)

B. The cognitive deficits in Criteria A1 and A2 each cause significant impairment in social or occupational functioning and represent a significant decline from a previous level of functioning.

C. Focal neurological signs and symptoms (e.g., exaggeration of deep tendon reflexes, extensor plantar response, pseudobulbar palsy, gait abnormalities, weakness of an extremity) or laboratory evidence indicative of cerebrovascular disease (e.g., multiple infarctions involving cortex and underlying white matter) that are judged to be etiologically related to the disturbance.

D. The deficits do not occur exclusively during the course of a delirium.

Code based on predominant features:

      290.41 With Delirium: if delirium is superimposed on the dementia

      290.42 With Delusions: if delusions are the predominant feature

      290.43 With Depressed Mood: if depressed moods (including presentations that meet full symptom criteria for a Major Depressive Episode) is the predominant feature. A separate diagnosis of Mood Disorder Due to a General Medical Condition is not given.

      290.40 Uncomplicated: if none of the above predominates in the current clinical presentation.

    Specify if:

        With Behavioral Disturbance

    Code note: Also code cerebrovascular condition on Axis III.

American Psychiatric Association Committee on Nomenclature and Statistics. *Diagnostic and Statistical Manual of Mental Disorders*. Washington DC: American Psychiatric Association, 1994.

DSMIV Diagnostic criteria for Delirium Due to . . .
(Indicate the General Medical Condition)

A. Disturbance of consciousness (i.e., reduced clarity of awareness of the environment) with reduced ability to focus, sustain, or shift attention.

B. A change in cognition (such as memory deficit, disorientation, language disturbance) or the development of a perceptual disturbance that is not better accounted for by a pre-existing, established, or evolving dementia.

C. The disturbance develops over a short period of time (usually hours to days) and tends to fluctuate during the course of the day.

D. There is evidence from the history, physician's examination, or laboratory findings that the disturbance is caused by the direct physiological consequences of a general medical condition.

Coding note: If delirium is superimposed on a preexisting Dementia of the Alzheimer's Type or Vascular Dementia, indicate the delirium by coding the appropriate subtype of the dementia, e.g., 290.3 Dementia of the Alzheimer's Type, With Late onset, With Delirium.

Coding note: Include the name of the general medical condition on Axis I, e.g., 293.0 Delirium Due to Hepatic Encephalopathy; also code the general medical condition on Axis III (see Appendix G for codes).

American Psychiatric Association Committee on Nomenclature and Statistics. *Diagnostic and Statistical Manual of Mental Disorders.* Washington DC: American Psychiatric Association, 1994.

COGNITIVE ASSESSMENT

Assessment of Delirium: The Confusion Assessment Method Instrument*

This instrument was validated in the inpatient setting where most delirium is generally diagnosed. However, it may have utility in the outpatient setting as well.

Characteristic	Descriptive Terms
Acute onset	Is there an acute change in mental status from patient's baseline?
Inattention	Did the patient have difficulty focusing attention, was easily distracted, or have difficulty keeping track of what was being said? Did this behavior, if present, fluctuate during the interview?
Disorganized thinking	Was the patient's thinking disorganized or incoherent, such as rambling or irrelevant conversation, unclear or illogical flow of ideas, or unpredictable switching from subject to subject?
Level of consciousness	Overall how would you rate this patient's level of consciousness? Alert (normal), hyperalert (startled easily, hypersenstive to environment), lethargic (easily aroused), stupor (difficult to arouse), coma.
Disorientation	Was the patient disoriented at any time during the interview, such as thinking that he/she was somewhere else, misjudging time of day, unable to identify present location?
Memory impairment	Did the patient exhibit any memory problems during the interview, such as inability to remember recent events or instructions?
Perceptual disturbances	Did the patient have any evidence of perceptual disturbances, such as hallucinations, illusions or misinterpretations?
Psychomotor agitation	At any time during the interview, did the patient have an unusually increased level of motor activity, such as restlessness, tapping fingers, or frequent sudden changes in position?
Psychomotor retardation	At any time during the interview, did the patient have an unusually decreased level of motor activity, such as sluggishness, staying in one position for a long time, staring into space, moving very slowly.
Altered sleep-wake cycle	Did the patient have evidence of disturbance of the sleep wake cycle, such as excessive daytime sleepiness with insomnia at night?

	Diagnostic Algorithm
Feature 1. **Acute Onset** **and Fluctuating Course**	Is there evidence of an acute change in mental status from the patient's baseline? Did the abnormal behavior fluctuate during the day?
Feature 2. **Inattention**	Did the patients have difficulty focusing attention?
Feature 3. **Disorganized Thinking**	Was the patient's thinking disorganized or incoherent?
Feature 4. **Altered Level** **of Consciousness**	Overall, how would you rate the patient's level of consciousness?

The Confusion Assessment Method Instrument

The diagnosis of delirium by the Confusion Assessment Method requires the presence of Features 1 and 2 and either 3 or 4.

★ Adapted from: Inouye, S.K., *et al*. Clarifying confusion: the confusion assessment method. *Ann Intern Med*. 1990; **113**: 941-948.

COGNITIVE ASSESSMENT DATABASE

The purpose of this tool is to assist the examiner in the evaluation of the patient with cognitive impairment and to direct the examiner towards the most likely diagnosis. The tool compiles a database for the evaluation of dementia. The diagnosis should be determined according to DSMIV criteria.

A. Symptoms

____ Memory loss   ____ Anxiety/Agitation
____ Forgets recent events   ____ Paranoid
____ Forgets things just said   ____ Delusions
____ Forgets names of people   ____ Hallucinations
____ Forgets words/names of objects   ____ Wanderings
____ Can't understand what is read   ____ Disruptive behaviour
____ Can't follow instructions   ____ Incontinence
____ Confused about date or place   ____ Gets lost
____ Can't do simple calculations   ____ Perseverates
     ____ Forgets how to do things

B. History

____ Hypertension   ____ Depression
____ Stroke   ____ Other Psychiatric Dx.
____ TIA

C. Onset of Symptoms

____ Recent (days to weeks)
____ Longer duration (months to years)
____ Uncertain

D. Progression of Symptoms

____ Rapid
____ Gradual
____ Stepwise
____ Uncertain

COGNITIVE ASSESSMENT(continued)

E. Other Significant Medical Conditions

1.	6.
2.	7.
3.	8.
4.	9.
5.	10.

F. Medication Review

1.	6.
2.	7.
3.	8.
4.	9.
5.	10.

G. Functional Status

ADL score _____   IADL score _____

H. Physical Examination

1. Blood pressure ___ / ___

2. Neurological Examination

state of consciousness? waxing and waning _____ alert _____
focal neurologic signs (document):
signs of Parkinsonism?

3. Gait:

4. Urinary incontinence? yes _____ no _____

I. Testing Examinations

1. Mini-Mental Status Examination   _____

2. Hachinski's or Loeb's Modified Ischemic Score _____

3. Geriatric Depression Scale _____

J. Diagnostic Studies as indicated

____	complete blood count	____	Electrolytes
____	liver functions tests	____	thyroid function tests (TSH)
____	sedimentation rate	____	Calcium
____	VDRL	____	B12/folate
____	chest X-ray	____	electrocardiogram
____	CT Head	____	LP
____	EEG	____	urinanalysis
____	Audiology/ Ophthamology	____	MRI

K. Diagnosis

____   Probable Alzheimer's type dementia

____   Vascular dementia

____   Mixed dementia

____   Potentially reversible cause of dementia (describe)

____   Depression

____   Delirium

____   Other psychiatric disease (describe)

If indicated, consult geriatrician, geriatric psychiatry, psychology (particularly for psychometrics), or neurology

Completed by _____

SOCIAL ASSESSMENTS

ASSESSMENT OF CAREGIVER STRESS

Significance of Problem

Informal caregiving, providing care for a relative or friend, involves many activities. Responsibilities can range from telephone calls and visits to check the older adult's status to the actual provision of physical care and management of problematic behaviors. More than 80% of care to older adults in the community is delivered by family members, often women, a majority of whom are also employed and may have nuclear family members, such as children, of their own.

Caregiving responsibilities cause employees to reduce hours worked or terminate employment and impact on other family obligations and relationships. The burden of caregiving can result in stress related illnesses. In some cases, caregiving is the responsibility of an aging spouse or sibling. In these situations, the individual fulfills the role of caregiver while dealing with his or her own functional decline.

Caregiver stress may contribute to institutionalization if the caregiver can no longer provide adequate care. In addition, it is a primary risk factor for elder neglect or abuse.

Assessment of Problem

A comprehensive functional assessment of the older adult helps to formulate a plan for the patient as well as the caregiver. Obtain information about formal and informal support systems already in place. Acknowledge that caregiver stress is common and ask direct questions about the caregiver's abilities to deal with the current situation. Remain objective and nonjudgmental.

Treatment and Management

Interventions to increase patient's functional level can lower intensity of caregiving.

The introduction of support systems into the patient's plan of care and education of caregiver about stress reduction strategies are valuable interventions to lessen caregiver burden. Social services can refer patients to community agencies for assistance with instrumental activities of daily living and activities of daily living. These resources may include home health aid/homemaker services, adult day care, mobile meals, transportation services and respite care. Private case managers can be employed to oversee responsibility for implementation of plan of care.

Education and counseling for the caregiver can occur in a support group environment and/or employee assistance program. Printed materials will help to reinforce the learning process. Encourage the caregiver to incorporate good health practices, such as proper nutrition, adequate sleep, exercise and recreation into his/her daily routine.

Acknowledge the family member's significant contribution to the patient's overall plan of care.

CAREGIVER ASSESSMENT

The purpose of this tool is to identify those caregivers who may be struggling unduly in their role as the primary care provider and to begin to identify methods of offering assistance that will alleviate some of the stessors.

Primary Caregiver:

Relation to Patient:

	YES/NO
1. Does the caregiver feel inconvenienced in their present role?	
2. Has the caregiver's health suffered because of their responsibilities toward the patient?	
3. Does the caregiver complain of physical hardships in caring for the patient?	
4. Does the caregiver feel confined or imprisoned in the home, and unable to have any private life?	
5. Has the caregiver's family had to make major adjustments in adapting to their new role?	
6. Has the caregiver had to change their life plans or feel as if they have lost control of their life?	
7. Does the caregiver feel the time needed to care for the patient is excessive?	
8. Does the patient display disruptive, embarrassing or upsetting behavior?	
9. Has the caregiver had to make employment changes in order to accommodate their new role?	
10. Is the caregiver under new financial constraints?	
11. Does the caregiver feel overwhelmed in their role?	

If a "YES" response is obtained to any question, consult Social Worker. If appropriate, consult Elder Abuse Team or Adult Protective Services in community.

Completed by _____

ASSESSMENT FOR ELDER ABUSE

Significance of Problem

It is estimated that over one million cases of elder abuse, an intentional harmful act toward an older adult, occur annually. Most instances of elder abuse are recurring events rather than a single episode. Consequences of abuse can be both physiologically and psychologically devastating to the older adult.

Cases of elder abuse are frequently unreported because of the victim's fear of retaliation, shame or desire to protect the abuser. In addition, inconsistencies among state governments regarding the definition of elder abuse and mandates for reporting cases make it difficult to assess magnitude of problem nationally.

Etiology

Factors which place an older adult at risk for elder abuse include:
- emotional impairment of the caregiver, especially drug or alcohol abuse
- history of violence within the family structure
- older adult's increasing dependency on caregiver due to physical or cognitive impairments
- stress, especially stress due to overwhelming caregiver responsibilities and stress due to financial problems.

Diagnosis

Medical History

The health care professional must remain nonjudgmental while obtaining the medical history that possibly relates to elder abuse. In addition, the interviewer should plan to spend some time alone with the patient. Begin the history with non-threatening questions, such as, "Tell me how you spend your day?' before direct ones regarding potential abuse. Be alert for inconsistencies in the reported history or between history and physical findings. Ask specific questions about the situation surrounding injuries.

Frequent transfer of care among health care providers and health care facilities or frequent missed appointments should be a signal for concern. Elicit information regarding the patient's level of functioning and the presence of formal and informal support systems involved in the patient's care.

Physical Exam

Observe interactions between patient and family members. Perform a functional assessment. Assess mental function and emotional state. Refer to the following table for classifications of elder abuse and clinical indicators to be alert for during the assessment process.

Type of abuse	Explanation of Terms	Clinical indicators
Physical	Infliction of physical pain or injury e.g., pushing, shoving, beating, inflicting burns; restraining; sexual assault; withholding medication, food or other necessities.	welts, burns, fractures, bruises, malnutrition or dehydration without obvious medical cause; poor personal hygiene; decubitus ulcers; trauma to genitalia; inappropriate medication use.
Psychological	Infliction of mental anguish by verbal insults, threats, patronizing comments, isolation.	low self esteem, paranoia, excessive fear, tearfulness, withdrawal, depression observed in the patient's behavior; caregiver behaviors: harsh tone of voice, discouraging communication with patient, disinterest in patient's condition.
Financial	Illegal or unethical exploiting by using funds, property or other assets of an older adult for personal gain e.g., pressure for older adult to relinquish assets, irresponsible handling of older adult's financial assets.	unfilled medication prescriptions, unpaid bills, sudden sale of property, unauthorized bank withdrawals.
Neglect	Intentional or unintentional failure to help older adult with daily needs and/or medical needs - **includes self neglect.**	reports of being left alone, malnutrition or dehydration without medical cause, poor personal hygiene, inappropriate medication use, unsafe home environment.

Treatment and Management

The patient's safety has priority in establishing a treatment plan. If the patient is in immediate danger and able to utilize decision making skills, options to relocate the patient away from the abuse situation should be presented. Utilize the assistance of social worker from adult protective services to establish a site for relocation.

If the older adult is in immediate danger, but does not have decision making skills, adult protective services will be responsible for relocation of the older adult and implemention of guardianship process.

Report cases of elder abuse to legal authorities as mandated. Document physical findings carefully.

A multidisciplinary effort is required to address the needs of the older adult at risk for elder abuse. The primary care provider should diagnosis and treat reversible and irreversible causes of cognitive impairment. Social services will provide referrals to appropriate community services, home care and/or respite care to assist in meeting the daily living needs of the patient, while reducing caregiver burden. Recommendations for legal aid and nursing home placement may also be provided.

Counseling may be appropriate for both the patient and abuser. Participation in a support group may introduce a stressed family member/caregiver to concepts about appropriate caregiver skills and stress reducing techniques.

A home assessment by a visiting nursing service can identify potential risks for the older adult's safety in that environment and generate recommendations for assistive devices to facilitate daily care activities.

All health care professionals in contact with older adults at risk for elder abuse need to assume a proactive role in teaching older adults and their caregivers about the aging process, available community resources and the normal progression of existing health conditions. This information will help both recipient of care and caregiver to establish realistic goals to meet the needs of the older adult.

ASSESSMENT FOR POTENTIAL OF ABUSE OR NEGLECT

The purpose of this tool is to identify those individuals and families who may, knowingly or unknowingly, be placing themselves into a situation where abuse or neglect of the patient may occur. It is not meant to give an absolute score, but rather to highlight areas of potential concern.

	Presence of Risks
A. CHARACTERISTICS OF THE PATIENT	
1. Female	
2. Advanced age	
3. Dependent	
4. Alcohol abuse	
5. Intergenerational conflict	
6. Internalizer	
7. Excessive loyalty	
8. Stoicism	
9. Isolation	
10. Impairment	
11. Provocative behavior	
12. Past abuse/neglect	
a. Physical	
b. Sexual	
c. Psychological	
d. Financial/material	
e. Neglect	

	Presence of Risks
B. CHARACTERISTICS OF THE CAREGIVER	
1. Alcohol use	
2. Medication/drug abuser	
3. Dementia/ confusion	
4. Mental/emotional illness	
5. Caregiving inexperience	
6. Economically troubled	
7. Abused as a child	
8. Stressed	
9. Unengaged outside of the home	
10. Blamer	
11. Unsympathetic	
12. Lacks understanding	
13. Unrealistic expectations	
14. Economically dependent	
15. Hypercritical	

ASSESSMENT FOR POTENTIAL OF ABUSE OR NEGLECT (continued)

C. CHARACTERISTICS OF THE FAMILY SYSTEM	
1. Lack of family support	
2. Caregiving reluctance	
3. Overcrowding	
4. Isolation	
5. Marital conflict	
6. Economic pressures	
7. Intra-family problems	
8. Desire for institutionalization	
9. Disharmony in shared responsibility	

D. CONGRUITY OF PERCEPTIONS BETWEEN PATIENT AND (POTENTIAL) CAREGIVER

1. Quality of past relationship

   a. Perception of the patient

   b. Perception of the caregiver

2. Quality of present relationship

   a. Perception of patient

   b. Perception of caregiver

3. Preferred placement location

   a. Perception of the patient

   b. Perception of the caregiver

4. Ideal placement location

   a. Perception of the patient

   b. Perception of the caregiver

E. IMPRESSION OF THE POTENTIAL FOR ABUSE OR NEGLECT:

If a potential for abuse or neglect of the patient is identified, or other areas of concern are noted, contact Social Worker or other services as appropriate.

Completed by _____

Adapted from: Kosberg, J.I. Preventing elder abuse: identification of high risk factors prior to placement decisions. *Gerontologist* 1988; **28** :43–50.

DETECTION OF ELDER ABUSE AND NEGLECT

A. HISTORY

____ 1. Pattern of physician or hospital hopping

____ 2. Unexplained delay in seeking treatment

____ 3. Series of missed medical appointments

____ 4. Previous unexplained injuries

____ 5. Explanation of past injuries inconsistent with findings

____ 6. Previous reports of similar injuries

____ 7. Patient appears fearful of family member

____ 8. Patient appears reluctant to respond when questioned

____ 9. Patient and caregiver/family members provide conflicting accounts of incident

____ 10. Family member is indifferent or angry towards patient and refuses to provide necessary assistance

____ 11. Family member appears overly concerned with costs of medical care and services

____ 12. Family member seeks to prevent the patient from interacting privately or speaking openly with health care provider

____ 13. Family member appears concerned about a particular patient problem but not the patient's overall health

____ 14. Unexplained or sudden inability to pay bills, purchase food or personal care items

____ 15. Extraordinary interest by family member in the patient's assets

____ 16. Excessive fears, withdrawal, resignation, agitation, apathy or ambivalence

B. PHYSICAL EXAMINATION

1. Unexplained fractures, welts, lacerations, punctures
2. Burns in unusual location, or of an unusual type or shape
3. Bruises in symmetrical or grouped pattern, or of a similar shape
4. Torn, stained, or bloody underclothing
5. Pain, itching, bruising, or bleeding in the genital region
6. Unexplained venereal disease or genital infections
7. Evidence of dehydration
8. Evidence of malnutrition or food deprivation
9. Hypo/hyperthermia due to environmental exposure
10. Inadequate personal hygiene
11. Inappropriate clothing for the season
12. Decubitus ulcers
13. Unexpected or unexplained deterioration of health
14. Unexplained evidence of medication mismanagement

Completed by _____

C. ASSESSMENT   _____ At risk _____ Not at risk

If any one or combination of these factors suggests the possibility of abuse or neglect (whether it is physical, sexual, psychological, or material), contact the Elder Abuse Team or Adult Protective Services Agency in community.

INSTITUTIONALIZATION RISK ASSESSMENT★

The purpose of this tool is to evaluate the aged in terms of their needs for institutionalization or their needs for community resources in terms of domiciliary care, group homes, day hospitals, etc.

For each item, circle the appropriate number and tally total score.

A. PHYSICAL CONDITION

1. Eyesight

0   a. Good enough to watch TV, read, do needlework, etc.
–3   b. Distinguishes faces
–10   c. Sees light only

2. Hearing

0   a. Good
–3   b. Hears only loud voices
–5   c. Deaf

3. Mobility

0   a. Fully mobile, dresses, carries parcels, rides buses, etc.
–3   b. Uses cane (or should) or is dependent upon fixtures
–15   c. Requires support in excess of a single cane

4. Cardiopulmonary Function

0   a. No restrictions
–3   b. Can manage 1 flight of stairs or 1 city block
–20   c. Partially or totally bed–ridden

5. Diet

0   a. No restrictions
     b. Normal
–3   c. Restrictions

B. MENTAL CONDITION

1. Disorientation

0   a. None
–3   b. Time
–15   c. Person and/or place

2. Delusions

0   a. None

–3   b. Mild–Severe Suspiciousness

–10 c. Overt

3. Memory Loss

0   a. None

–3   b. Benign

–20 c. Malignant

4. Energy and Drive

0   a. Normal

–5   b. Hypoactive or hyperactive

5. Judgement

0   a. Intact

–5   b. Impaired

6. Hallucinations

0   a. None

–10 b. Auditory and/ or visual

C. FUNCTIONAL ABILITIES

+2   A. Reads and writes letters

+5   B. Able to use telephone

+5   C. Able to bank and shop

+7   D. Able to prepare simple meals and bake

+5   E. Washes, dresses, and toilets self without assistance

+7   F. Uses public transportation

+10 G. Able to take own medication and follow diet

D. SUPPORT FROM THE COMMUNITY

+2   1. Ethnic compatibility

+10 2. If living alone, can get support and help from a reliable relative, friend, or neighbor

+5   3. Able to shop at a reliable grocery (with delivery services)

       4. Available supportive and recreational facilities:

+2   a. clubs geared to the aged

+1   b. church, synagogue

+1   c. library

+1   d. park, shopping center, restuarant, movies

5. Geographic availability of:

+2	a. public health nurses, VNS, etc.
+2	b. Meals–on–Wheels services
+2	c. homemaker services
+2	d. friendly visitors
+2	e. hospital with emergency and clinic facilities
+2	f. public transportation

E.   LIVING QUARTERS

+3	1. Elevator service
+3	2. Living on ground floor

F.   RELATIVES AND FRIENDS

+5	1. Not married but lives with compatible and helpful friend or relative
0	2. Lives with incompatible relative, friend, or spouse
+10	3. Lives with able and compatible spouse

G.   FINANCIAL SITUATION

+5	1. Totally independent
+3	2. Dependent on helpful relative
0	3. Dependent primarily on governmental sources of income

TOTAL NEGATIVE SCORE: _____

TOTAL POSITIVE SCORE: _____

FINAL SCORE: _____

If score is <20, patient will likely require institutionalization

If score is 20-40, patient will need assistance to exist in the community successfully

If score is >40, patient will likely need no outside help and can usually function independently

Completed by _____

★ Adapted from: Grauer, H., Birnbom, B.A. A geriatric functional rating scale to determine the need for institutional care. *J. Am. Geriatr. Soc.* 1975; **23**: 472-476.©1975 Grauer and Birnbom.

ADVANCED DIRECTIVES IN THE CARE OF THE ELDERLY

Significance

Recent studies have demonstrated that most patients have inadequate or no discussions concerning their advanced directives. Advanced directives provide the elderly patient with the opportunity to control their destiny and have their wishes for treatment respected and followed. When there is discordance among patients, caregivers, and providers about care, unwanted and sometimes inappropriate treatments are provided, conflicts increase, and so do costs. In the end, the patient loses control of the end of their life, their wishes may not be met, and the patient suffers. Numerous methods for increasing the opportunities for obtaining advanced directives and insuring compliance with them in the outpatient and inpatient settings have been suggested, but ultimately, it is the provider's responsibility to initiate discussions of advanced directives as part of routine patient care, particularly in the frail elderly, and to insure that advanced directives are understood and completed by the patient and caregivers.

Assessment

Various tools exist which attempt to organize aspects of advanced directives into usable formats. Advanced directives may include a living will, a durable power of attorney for health care, a health care proxy, a medical directive and a values history. All of these are far more inclusive and usable for both the patient, caregivers and the provider than the simple "do not resuscitate" order which addresses a single issue at the very end of life. Informal discussions around these sometimes sensitive issues may be preferred to an organized format. It is frequently surprising to the provider to learn that the primary obstacle to such frank and detailed discussions are often in the provider's mind, not in the patient's, who often greatly appreciates such discussions and finds relief in them. Legal aspects of advanced directives also vary considerably among the states, and providers need to be aware of their own state's legal rules regarding advanced directives.

Management

Advanced directives are most optimally obtained in the ambulatory care setting when patients are not acutely ill and under duress. Although the stability of directives obtained in the ambulatory care setting may change, prior information is nevertheless crucial in establishing a therapeutic rapport with patients on sensitive issues. Periodic confirmation of patients' wishes assist in obtaining stable and confirmed directives. Documentation of patients' wishes, and documentation of where formal documents such as living wills and health care proxies are held are important during times of acute illness when they are most needed. Living wills and a values history frame patients' wishes in context, while medical directives document patient wishes on specific treatments such as artificial feeding and hydration, dialysis, antibiotics, mechanical ventilation, hospitalization and other treatments. Health care proxies avoid the disadvantages of attempt to define treatments out of context, and give power to designated caregivers to provide decision making capacity on all issues on behalf of the values of the patient. Counselling patients on the process of how advanced directive documents and proxies are used in the clinical setting is important in insuring that the wishes of the patient can be implemented through their documents or proxies.

Discussion of advanced directives often take time. It is not always required that the discussion be held between the physician and the patient. Social workers and case managers may also be involved in obtaining advanced directives, at least in the context of providing appropriate legal documents such as proxies, but also in counselling. Whether advanced directives save costs at the end of life remains an issue for clinical investigation. Nevertheless, the empowerment of individuals to control their destiny and quality of life at the end of life, whatever their values, is the primary goal of advanced directives and should be respected and implemented for all patients whenever possible.

PALLIATIVE CARE PLANNING

The purpose of this tool is to assist the patient and caregiver in the development of a set of guidelines for the provision of care at the end of life.

1. Does the patient have a terminal diagnosis (i.e. is the patient's lifespan likely to be 6 months or less)?

    YES _____   NO _____

    A. If "Yes", has the patient designated any medical directives?

        YES _____   NO _____

        If "Yes", be certain that they are documented on the medical record.
        If "No", proceed to 2.

    B. If "No", has the patient designated any medical directives?

        YES _____   NO _____

        If "Yes", be certain that they are documented on the medical record.
        If "No", proceed to 2.

2. At the minimum the following Medical Directives should be discussed with the patient and/or surrogates/caregiver(s):

    A. Has a durable power of attorney been appointed? Yes No
        If "Yes", who?

    B. 1) Does the patient have a Living Will?   Yes No
        If "Yes", is a copy available?

       2) Does the patient have a health care proxy?   Yes No
        If "Yes", is a copy available?

        If "yes", who is the surrogate?

TERMINAL CARE PLANNING

C. Cardiopulmonary resuscitation   Yes   No

D. Mechanical ventilation   Yes   No

E. Artificial nutrition and hydration   Yes   No

F. Major surgery   Yes   No

G. Minor surgery   Yes   No

H. Kidney dialysis   Yes   No

I. Chemotherapy   Yes   No

J. Invasive diagnostic tests   Yes   No

K. Blood or blood products   Yes   No

L. Antibiotics   Yes   No

M. Simple diagnostic tests   Yes   No

N. Pain medications   Yes   No

O. Organ donation   Yes   No

P. Autopsy   Yes   No

Q. Other _____

     Specifics should be noted in the medical record

Completed by _____

Adapted from: Emanuel, L., Emmanuel, E., The Medical Directive. *J. Amer. Med.Assoc.* 1989; **261**: 3288-3289.

THE VALUES HISTORY

This Values History is intended to serve as a set of specific directives of care to be appended to my Living Will. It is to be used in health care circumstances when I may be unable to voice my preferences. Like my Living Will, these directives are to be made a part of the medical record and used under the "terminal condition" terminology of the Living Will.

I. VALUES SECTION

There are a number of values that are relevant to decisions about terminal treatment and care. This section of the Values History invites you to identify your most important values.

A. Basic Life Values

Perhaps the most basic values in this context concern length of life versus quality of life. Which of the following two statements is the most important to you?

1. I want to live as long as possible, regardless of the quality of life that I experience.
2. I want to preserve a good quality of life, even if this means that I may not live as long.

B. Quality of Life Values

There are many values that help us to define for ourselves the quality of life that we want to live. The following list contains some of the most common of those. Review this list (and feel free to add to it) indicating the values that are important to your definition of quality of life.

1. I want to maintain my capacity to think clearly.
2. I want to feel safe and secure.
3. I want to avoid unnecessary pain and suffering.
4. I want to be treated with respect.
5. I want to be treated with dignity when I can no longer speak for myself.
6. I do not want to be an unnecessary burden on my family.
7. I want to be able to make my own decisions.
8. I want to experience a comfortable dying process.
9. I want to be able to be with my loved ones before I die.
10. I want to leave good memories of me to my loved ones.
11. I want to be treated in accord with my religious beliefs and traditions.
12. I want respect shown for my body after I die.
13. I want to help others by making a contribution to medical education and research.
14. Other values:

C. Ranking Values : Of the above values, which three are the most important to you.

II. DIRECTIVES SECTION: Circle as appropriate with Initials and Date

1. I DO/DO NOT wish to undergo resuscitation. Why?

2. I DO/DO NOT wish to be placed on a ventilator. Why?

3. I DO/DO NOT wish to have an endotracheal tube utilized in order to perform items 1 and 2. Why?

4. I DO/DO NOT wish to have total parenteral nutrition administered for my nutrition. Why?

5. I DO/DO NOT wish to have intravenous medication and hydration administered; however, I understand that intravenous hydration to alleviate discomfort and pain medication will not be withheld from me if I so request them. Why?

6. I DO/DO NOT wish to have all medications for the treatment of my illness continued; however, I understand that pain medication will not be withheld from me if I so request it. Why?

7. I DO/DO NOT wish to be placed on a dialysis machine. Why?

8. I DO/DO NOT wish to have an autopsy performed in order to determine the cause(s) of my death. Why?

Completed by _____   Date: _____

Adapted from: Doukas, D.J., McCullough, L.B., The values history: the evaluation of the patient's values and advance directives. *J. Fam. Practice.* 1991; **32:** 145-153.

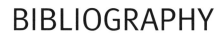

BIBLIOGRAPHY

BIBLIOGRAPHY

Comprehensive Geriatric Assessment

General Reviews

Deyo, R., *et al.* Editors: The future of geriatric assessment, *J. Amer. Geriatr. Soc.* Volume 39, supplement. 1991. Complete supplement to volume 39 is devoted to geriatric assessment.

Engelhardt, J.B., *et al.* The effectiveness and efficiency of outpatient geriatric evaluation and management. *J. Amer. Geriatr. Soc.* 1996 **44**: 847–856.

Fillit, H. and Capello, C., Making geriatric assessment an asset to your primary care practice. *Geriatrics* 1994. **49**: 27–35.

Moore, A.A. and Siu, A.L. Screening for common problems in ambulatory elderly: clinical confirmation of a screening instrument. *Am. J. Med.* 1996 **100**: 438–443.

Scanemeo, A.M. and Fillit, H. Housecalls: a practical guide to seeing the patient at home. *Geriatrics* 1995 **50**: 33–39.

Stuck A.E, Siu A.L, Wieland D., *et al.* Comprehensive geriatric assessment: a meta–analysis., of controlled trials. *Lancet* 1993 **142**: 1032–1036.

Geriatric Assessment Units

Epstein, A.M., Hall, J.A., Besdine, R., Cumella, E.Jr., Feldstein, M., McNeil, J. and Rowe, J.W. The emergence of geriatric assessment units: the new technology of geriatrics. *Ann. Intern. Med.* 1987 **106**: 299–303.

Fillit, H., Challenges for acute care geriatric inpatient units operating under current Medicare Prospective Payment. *J. Amer. Geriatr. Soc.* 1994 **42**: 553–558.

Inouye, S.K., *et al.* The Yale geriatric care program: a model of care to prevent functional decline in hospitalized elderly patients. *J. Amer. Geriatr. Soc.* 1993 **41**: 1345–1352.

Palmer, R.M., Landefeld, S. and Kowal, J. A medical unit for the acute care of the elderly. *J. Amer. Geriatr. Soc.* 1994 **42**: 545–552.

Geriatrics and Managed Care

Kramer, A.M., Fox, P.D. and Morgenstern, N. Geriatric care approaches in health maintenance organizations. *J. Amer. Geriatr. Soc.* 1992 **40**: 1055-1067.

Friedman, B. and Kane, R.L. HMO medical directors' perceptions of geriatric practice in Medicare HMOs. *J. Amer. Geriatr. Soc.* 1993 **41**: 1144-1149.

Fillit, H. Geriatrics and health care reform: opportunities in managed care for preserving excellence in the care of the elderl., *Ann. N.Y. Acad. Sci.* 1994 **729**: 331-339.

Lopez, L. Improving care for the elderly. *Healthplan* 1996 **37**: 39-46.

von Sternberg, T. Geriatrics as a value-added service within an HMO. *Clin. Geriatr.* 1995 **3**: 42-45.

High Risk Screening

Boult, C., *et al.* Screening elders for risk of hospital admission. *J. Amer. Geriatric. Soc.* 1993 **41**: 811-817.

Pacala, J.T., Boult, C. and Boult, L. Predictive validity of a questionnaire that identifies older persons at risk for hospital admission. *J. Amer. Geriatr. Soc.* 1995 **43**: 374-377.

Case Management

Aliotta, S.L. Components of a sucessful case management program. *Managed Care Quart.* 1996 **4**: 38-45.

Warren, B.H., Puls, T. and Fogelstrom-DeZeeuw, P. Cost-effectiveness of case management experiences of a University managed health care organization. *Am. J. Med. Qual.* 1996 **11**: 173-178.

Alcoholism

Alcohol abuse and dependence. In: *The Merck Manual of Geriatrics*, ed. by Abrams, W.B., Beers, M.H., Berkow, R. 2nd. ed., Merck Research Laboratories, Whitehouse Station, 1995, Chapter 99, pp 1245-1248.

Fulop, G., Rheinhardt, J., Strain, J.J., Paris, B., Miller, M. and Fillit, H., Alcohol abuse and depression in frail elderly outpatient., *J. Amer. Geriatr. Soc.* 1993 **41**: 737-741.

Slezer, M.L. The Michigan Alcoholism Screening Test: The quest for a new diagnostic instrument. *Amer. J. Psychiat.* 1991 **12**: 1653-1658.

Weatherford, W. Alcohol abuse in the aging population: a silent epidemic. *Clin. Geriatr.* 1996 **4**: 56-80.

Caregiver Stress

Andolsek, *et al.* Caregivers and elderly relatives. *Arch. Intern. Med.* 1988 **148**: 2177.

Barusch, A.S. Problems and coping strategies of elderly spouse caregivers. *Gerontologist* 1988 **28**: 677-685.

Green, J.G. *et al.* Relatives stress scale. *Age and Aging* 1982 **11**: 121.

Kosberg, *et al.* Components of burden: interventive implications. *Gerontologist* 1990 **30**: 236.

Smith, G.C., Smith, M.F. and Toseland R.W. Problems identified by family caregivers in counselling. *Gerontologist* 1991 **31**: 15-21.

Waltman, R. Supporting the caregiver's role. *Geriatric Consultan*t 1993 **March-April**,14-19.

Zarit, S. and Whitlach, C. Problems identified by intermediaries with caregivers: a re-analysis. *Gerontologist* 1991 **31**: 9-13.

Cognitive Impairment

American Psychiatric Association Committee on Nomenclature and Statistics *DSM IV. Diagnostic and Statistical Manual of Mental Disorders*, Washington, DC: American Psychiatric Association, 1994.

Delirium:

Albert, M.A. *et al.* The delirium symptom interview: an interview for the detection of delirium symptoms in hospitalized patients. *J. Geriatr. Psych. Neurol.* 1992 **5**: 14.

Inouye, S.K. The dilemna of delirium: clinical and research controversies regarding diagnosis and evaluation of delirium in hospitalized elderly medical patients. *Am. J. Med.* 1994 **97**: 278.

Inouye, S.K., van Dyck, C.H., Alessi, C.A., Balkin, S., Siegal, A.P. and Horvitz, R.I. Clarifying confusion: the confusion assessment method; a new method for detection of delirium". *Ann. Intern. Med.* 1990 **113**: 941-948.

Dementia

Fillit, H. Future therapeutic developments of estrogen use. *J. Clin. Pharmacol.* 1995 **35**: s25–s28.

Folstein, M., Folstein, S. and McHugh, P.R. Mini-Mental State: a practical method of grading the cognitive state of patients for the clinician *J. Psychiat. Res.* 1975 **12**: 189–198.

Gledmacher, D.S. and Whitehouse, P.J. Evaluation of dementia. *N. Engl. J. Med.* 1996 **335**: 330–336.

Hachinski, V.C. Vascular dementia: a radical redefinition. *Dementia* 1994 **5**: 130 .

Lusis, S.A., Hydo, B. and Clark, L. Nursing assessment of mental status in the elderly. *Geriatr. Nursing* 1993 **14**: 255–259.

McKeith, I.G., Fairbairn, A.F., Perry, R.H. and Thompson, P. The clinical diagnosis and misdiagnosis of senile dementia of Lewy Body Type (SDLT). *Brit. J. Psychiat.* 1994 **165**: 324–332.

Loeb, C. and Gandolfo, C. Diagnostic evaluation of degenerative and vascular dementia. *Stroke* 1983 **14**: 399.

Mace, N.L. and Rabins, P.V. 1991 *The 36-Hour Day*. Baltimore: The Johns Hopkins University Press.

Schneider, L.S. and Tariot, P.N. Emerging drugs for Alzheimer's disease: mechanisms of action and prospects for cognitive enhancing medications. *Med. Clin. N. Amer.* 1994 **78**: 911.

Skoog, I., Nilsson, L., Palmertz, B., Andreasson, L. and Svanborg, A. A population based study of dementia in 85 year olds. *N. Engl. J. Med.* 1993 **328**: 153–158.

Tangelos, E.G., *et al.* The Mini-Mental State Examination in general medical practice: clinical utility and acceptance. *Mayo Clinic Proceedings* 1996 **71**: 829–837.

Depression

Butler, R.N., Lewis, M. and Sunderland, T. *Aging and Mental Health*; 4ed., New York, 1991. Macmillan Publishing Company.

desRosiers, G., Hodges, J.R. and Berrios, G. The neuropsychological differentiation of patients with very mild Alzheimer's disease and/or major depression. *J. Amer. Geriatr. Soc.* 1995 **43**: 1256–1263.

Slater, S.L. and Katz, I.R. Prevalence of depression in the aged: formal calculations versus clinical facts._ *J. Amer. Geriatr. Soc.* **43**: 78-79, 1995.

Yesavage, J., Brink, T.L., Rose, T.L., Lum, O., Huang, V., Adey, M. and Leirer, V.O. Development and validation of a geriatric depression screening scale: a preliminary report. *J. Psych. Res.* 1983 **17**: 37-49.

Elder Abuse and Neglect

Elder Abuse and Neglect. Council on Scientific Affairs. *J. Amer. Med. Assoc.* *1987* **257(7)** 966-971.

Conlin, M.M. Silent suffering: a case study of elder abuse and neglect. *J. Amer. Geriatr. Soc.* 1995 **43**: 1303-1308.

Kosberg, J.I. Preventing elder abuse: identification of high risk factors prior to placement decisions. *Gerontologist* 1988 **28**: 43.

Wolf, R.S. Elder abuse: ten years later. *J. Amer. Geriatr. Soc.* 1988 **36**: 758.

Yurkow, J. Elder abuse. *Trends in Health Care, Law and Ethics.* 1993. **8**: 60-62,

Falls

Nevitt, M.C., *et al.* Risk factors for recurrent nonsyncopal falls. *JAMA* 1989 **261**: 2663.

Rizzo, J.A., Baker, D.I. McAvay, G. and Tinetti, M.E. The cost-effectiveness of a multifactorial targeted prevention program for falls among community elderly persons. *Medical Care* 1996 **34**: 954-969.

Rodriquez, J.G., *et al.* A. A standardized instrument to assess hazards for falls in the home of older persons. *Accid. Anal. and Prev.* 1995 **27**: 625-631.

Rubenstein, L.Z. *et al.* The value of assessing falls in an elderly population; a randomized clinical trial. *Ann. Intern. Med.* 1990 **113**: 108.

Tideiskaar, R. and Fillit, H. Falls in the elderly, in: *Seizures and epilepsy in the elderly.* Rowan, A.J. and Ramsay, R.E. (eds.). 1997 Boston: Butterworth-Heinemann, pp. 87-110.

Fecal Incontinence

Dodge, *et al.* Fecal incontinence in elderly patient. *Post. Grad. Med.* 1988 **83**: 258-270.

Madoff, R.D., Williams, J.G., Caushaj, P.F. Fecal incontinence. *N. Engl. J. Med.* 1992 **326**: 1002–1007.

Sodeman, W.A., Saladin, T.A., Boyd, W.P. *Geriatric Gastroenterology* WB Saunders, 1989.

Feeding

Martin, A.W., Dietary management of swallowing disorders. *Dysphagia* 1991 **6**: 129–134.

Mendez, L. *et al.* Swallowing disorders in the elderly. *Clin. Geriatr. Med.* 1991 **7: 2**: 215–230.

Morley, J.E. Anorexia in older patients: its meaning and management . *Geriatrics* 1990 **45**: 59–66.

Functional Assessment

Fleming, K., Evans, J., Weber, D. and Chunka, D. Practical functional assessment of elderly persons: a primary care approach. *Mayo Clinic Proceedings* 1995 **70**: 890–910.

Katz, S., *et al.* Studies of illness in the aged: The index of ADL; a standardized measure of biological and psychosocial function. *J. Amer. Med. Assoc.* 1963 **185**: 914–919.

Katz, S. and Stroud, M.W. III Functional assessment in geriatrics. *J. Am.Geriatr. Soc.* 1989 **37**: 267–271.

Lawton, M.P. and Brody, E.M. Assessment of older people: self-maintaining and instrumental activity of older daily living. *Gerontologist* 1969 **9**: 179–186.

Narain, P., *et al.* Predictors of immediate and 6-month outcomes in hospitalized elderly patients: the importance of functional status. *J. Am.Geriat. Soc.* 1988 **36**: 775–783.

Gait Disorders/Immobility

Sudarsky, L. Gait disorders in the elderly. *N. Engl. J. Med.* 1990 **322**: 441–46.

Health Maintenance

Manton, K.G., Stallard, E. and Corder, L.S. Changes in morbidity and chronic disability in the US elderly. population: evidence from the 1982, 1984 and 1989 National Long Term Care Surveys. *J. Gerontol.* 1995 **50B**: S194–S204.

Scheitel, S.M., Fleming, K.C., Chutka, D.S. and Evans, J.M. Geriatric health maintenance. *Mayo Clin. Proc.* 1996 **71**: 289–302.

US Preventive Services Task Force. 1996 *Guide to Clinical Preventive Services*. Baltimore: Williams and Wilkins.

Hearing Impairment

Bess, F., Lichtenstein, M. and Logan S. Hearing impairment as determinant of function in the elderly. *J. Amer. Geriatr. Soc.* 1989 **37**: 123-128.

Fisch, L. and Brooks, D.N. Disorders of hearing. In: Brocklehurst, J.C., Tallis, R., and Fillit, H.M., (eds.), 1992: *Textbook of Geriatric Medicine and Gerontology,* 4ed., London, Churchill Livingstone, pp. 480.

Lichtenstein, M.J., Bess, F.H., Logan, S.A. Validation of screening tools for identifying hearing impaired elderly in primary care. *J. Amer. Med.Assoc.* 1988 **259**: 2875-2878.

Mulrow, C., *et al.* Quality of life changes and hearing impairment: results of a randomized trial. *Ann. Intern. Med.* 1990 **113**: 188-194.

Immunocompetence Assessment

Fillit, H. Clinical immunology of aging. *Rev. Clin. Gerontol.* 1994 **4**: 187-197.

Fillit, H.M. Practical evaluation of secondary immune deficiencies in the elderl., *Geriatrics* 1991 **46**: 70.

Mulvihill, M., Cohen, C., Martemucci, W., Taylor, B., Libow, L.S., Neufeld, R. and Fillit, H. Energy in the frail elderly is associated with an increased rate of infection and mortality. *Aging: Immunol. Infect. Dis.* 1995 **6**: 1-13.

Rosenzweig, R. and Fillit, H. Probable heterosexual transmission of AIDS in an aged woman. *J. Am.Geriatr. Soc.* 1992 **40**: 1261-1264.

Institutionalization Risk

Graner and Birnborn. A geriatric functional rating scale to determine the need for institutional care. *J. Amer. Geriatr. Soc.* 1975 **10**: 472-476.

Nutrition

Agraval, *et al.* Predictive ability of various nutritional variables for mortality in elderly people. *Am. J.Clin. Nutr.* 1988 **48**: 1173-8.

Lansey, S., Waslien, C., Mulvihill, M. and Fillit, H. The role of anthropometric assessment for malnutrition in the hospitalized frail elderly. *Gerontology* 1993 **39**: 346–353.

Morley, J.E. Why do physicians fail to recognize and treat malnutrition in older persons? *J. Amer. Geriatr. Soc.* 1991 **39**: 1139–1140.

Posner, B.M., *et al.* Nutrition and health risks in the elderly: The nutrition screening initiative. *Am. J. Public Health* 1993 **83**: 972–978.

Weinster, *et al.* A prospective evaluation of general medical patients during the course of hospitalization. *Am. J. Clin. Nutr.* 1979 **32**: 418–426.

Oral and Dental Assessment

Baum, B.J. (ed.) *Oral and dental problems in the elderly.* 1992 Philadelphia: W. B. Saunders Co.

Bush, L.A., Horenkamp, N., Morley, J.E. and Spiro, A.I. D-E-N-T-A-L: a rapid self-administered screening instrument to promote referrals for further evaluation in older adults. *J. Amer. Geriatr. Soc.* 1996 **44**: 979–981.

Osteoporosis

Abbott, T.A.I., Lawrence, B.J. and Wallach, S. Osteoporosis: the need for comprehensive treatment guidelines. *Clin. Therapeutics* 1996 1**8**: 127–149.

Francis, R.M. Bone aging, osteoporosis, and osteomalacia. In: Brocklehurst, J.C., Tallis, R. and Fillit, H.M., (eds.), 1992 *Textbook of Geriatric Medicine and Gerontology, 4ed.* London, Churchill Livingstone, pp. 769.

Riggs, B.L. and Melton, L.J. Involutional osteoporosis. *N. Engl. J. Med.* 1986 **314**: 1676–1686.

Palliative Care

Emanuel, L. and Emmanuel, E. The medical directive. *J. Amer. Med. Assoc.* 1989 **261**: 3288–3289.

Doukas, D.J. and McCullough, L.B. 1988 Assessing the values history of the elderly patient regarding critical and chronic care. In: *Handbook of Geriatric Assessment.* W. Reichel and J. Gallo, (eds.), Aspen Press, 1988, p.110.

Gillick, M.R. A broader role for advance medical planning. *Ann. Intern. Med.* 1995 **123**: 621 624.

Schonwetter, R.S. Care of the terminally patient. *Clin. Geriatr. Med.* Philadelphia: W.B. Saunders Company, **12**: 1996 .

Polypharmacy

Chutka, D.S., Evans, J.M., Fleming, K.C. and Mikkelson, K.G. Drug prescribing for elderly patients. *Mayo Clinic Proceedings* 1995 **70**: 685-693.

Kroenke, K., Polypharmacy: causes, consequences, and cure. *Am. J. Med.* 1985 **79**: 149-152.

Montamat, Cusack, S. and Cusack B. Overcoming problems with polypharmacy and drug misuse in the elderly. *Clin. Geriatr. Med.* **8**: 143-158.

Schmader, K. *et al.* Appropriateness of medication prescribing in ambulatory elderly patients. *J. Amer. Geriatr. Soc.* 1994 **42**: 1241-1247.

Pre-Operative Risk Assessment

Thomas, D.R., Ritchie, C.S. Preoperative assessment of older adults. *J. Amer. Geriatr. Soc.* 1995 **43**: 811-821.

Owens, W.D., Felts, J.A., Spitznagel, E.L. Jr. ASA Physical status classifications: A study of consistency of ratings. *Anesthesiology* 1978 **49:** 239.

Goldman, L. Cardiac risks and complication of non-cardiac surgery. *Ann. Intern. Med.* 1983 **98**: 504.

Goldman, L., *et al.* Multifactorial index of cardiac risk in non cardiac surgical procedure. *N. Engl. J. Med.* 1977 **297**: 845.

Detsky, AS, *et al.* Predicting complications in patients undergoing non-cardiac surgery. *J. Gen. Intern. Med.* 1986 **1:** 211-219.

Pressure Ulcers

Allman, R.M. Pressure ulcers among the elderly. *N. Engl. J. Med.* 1989 **320**: 850.

Bergstrom, N., *et al.* 1994 Treatment of pressure ulcers. clinical practice guidelines, U.S. Department of Health and Human Services. December.

Patterson, J. and Bennett, R. Prevention and treatment of pressure sores. *J. Amer. Geriatr. Soc.* 1995 **43**: 8.

Towey, A., *et al.* Validity and reliability of an assessment tool for pressure ulcer risk. *Decubitus* 1988 **1**: 40.

Rehabilitation

Martin, G.M., Prescribing physical and occupational therapy. *Mayo Clinic Proceedings* 1985 **36**: 510-518,

Mosqueda, L.A. Assessment of rehabilitation potential. *Clin. Geriatr. Med.* 1993 **9**: 689-704.

Weber., D.C, Fleming, K.C, and Evans, J.M., Rehabilitation of geriatric patients. *Mayo Clinic Proceedings* 1995 **70:** 1198-1204.

Sleep Disorder

Chien, N.T. Sleep disorders in the elderly. *Clin. Geriatr.* 1996 **4:** 44-62.

Prinz, P.N., Vitiello, M.V., Raskind, M.A. and Thorpy, M.J. Geriatrics: sleep disorders and aging. *N. Engl. J. Med.* 1990 **323**: 520-526.

Urinary Incontinence

Chutka, D.S., Fleming K.C, and Evans M.P. *et al.* Urinary incontinence in the elderly population. *Mayo Clinic Proceedings* 1996 **71**: 93-101.

Fantl, J. Newman, A., Kaschak, D., *et al.* March, 1996 Urinary Incontinence in Adults: Acute and Chronic Management. U.S. Department of Health and Human Services.

Ouslander, J., *et al.* Prospective evaluation of an assessment strategy for geriatric urinary incontinence. *J. Amer. Geriatr. Soc.* 1989 **37**: 715-724.

Visual Impairment

Brodie, S. Aging and disorders of the eye. In: Brocklehurst, J.C., Tallis, R., and Fillit, H.M., (eds.), 1992 *Textbook of Geriatric Medicine and Gerontology,* 4 ed., London, Churchill Livingstone, pp. 472.

Faye, E. and Stuen, C. 1992 *The Aging Eye and Low Vision.* The Lighthouse, Inc.

INDEX